ARTHRITIS DIET COOKBOOK FOR SENIORS

Nourishing, Anti-Inflammatory Recipes to Ease Joint Pain and Enhance Daily Living

Kingsley Klopp

To show our appreciation for your purchase, we're delighted to offer you these special bonuses as a heartfelt thank you.

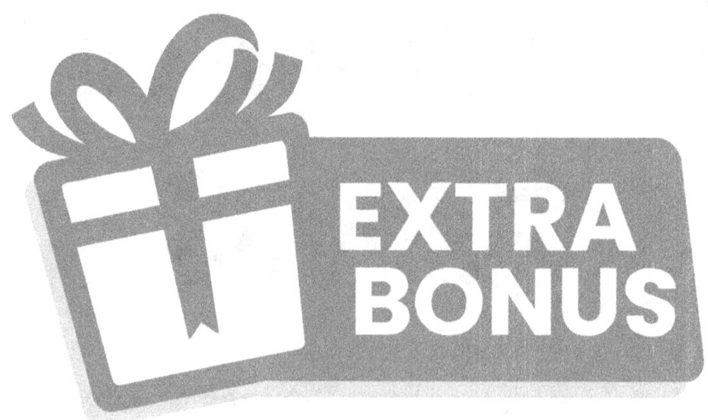

1. A Food Tracker Journal
2. Downloadable E-BOOK featuring full-color images of finished recipes

Table of Contents

Fish and Seafood Recipes

Vegetables

Soup and Stew Recipes

Important Note

This book is crafted with love and care, keeping in mind the diverse tastes and dietary needs of seniors who wish to nourish their bodies and soothe their joints through thoughtful, healthy eating. However, it's important to remember that each individual's journey with arthritis is unique, just like our taste in food! As such, while the recipes within these pages offer a foundation for an anti-inflammatory diet aimed at reducing arthritis symptoms, they are starting points. We encourage you to embrace the flexibility to modify these recipes according to your personal health requirements, dietary restrictions, and preferences. Feel free to substitute ingredients, adjust seasonings, or alter cooking methods to suit your taste and nutritional needs.

We understand that navigating dietary changes can sometimes be as challenging as dealing with arthritis itself. If you ever find yourself puzzled or uncertain about how to tailor these recipes to better suit your health conditions, or if a particular dietary change is suitable for you, please consult your healthcare provider. They can provide guidance that is specifically tailored to your health profile, ensuring that the dietary choices you make contribute positively to your arthritis management plan.

Please also be aware that the nutritional information provided alongside each recipe is approximate. Factors such as the brand of ingredients used, natural variability in fresh produce, and portion sizes can all influence the nutritional values. Therefore, use these numbers as a guide rather than an exact measurement. They are intended to help you make informed decisions about your eating habits, empowering you to take control of your diet in a way that benefits your overall health and arthritis symptoms.

Furthermore, If our cookbook has brought joy to your kitchen and table, we'd be thrilled to hear about your experiences in an Amazon review. On the flip side, if you stumble upon any hiccups while exploring our recipes, don't hesitate to get in touch at **kloppkingsley@gmail.com**. We're here to support your cooking journey every step of the way.

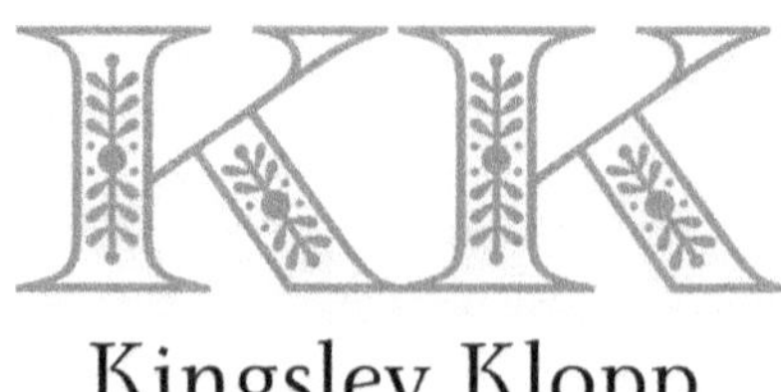

Kingsley Klopp

Introduction.

Imagine a morning where the simple joy of opening a jar, turning a doorknob, or walking to the mailbox isn't overshadowed by the piercing twinge of joint pain. Where each movement isn't a reminder of the arthritis that has tried to claim your golden years. This isn't just a hopeful daydream; it's a very real possibility, and it all begins with what's on your plate.

Welcome to the "**Arthritis Diet Cookbook for Seniors**," a culinary companion designed to empower you as you navigate the challenges of arthritis with wisdom and flavor. This book isn't just about meals; it's about reclaiming the vibrancy and vitality of your senior years, one delicious dish at a time. You might wonder how a cookbook can be so transformative. The answer lies in understanding the profound impact food has on our bodies, especially when dealing with chronic conditions like arthritis. Inflammation is a key contributor to the pain and stiffness you feel, and this cookbook focuses on foods that naturally combat this inflammation. It's about turning each meal into an opportunity for relief and prevention. But let's get something straight: this isn't your typical diet cookbook. We know that seniors like you have rich lives and discerning palates. You've savored decades of meals, from quick lunches in bustling city cafes to leisurely dinners at home with loved ones. You appreciate good food, and you deserve recipes that are not only healthy but also flavorful and satisfying. That's exactly what you'll find here: dishes that delight the taste buds while being gentle on the joints. As we age, our bodies change, and so do our nutritional needs. This cookbook is tailored specifically for seniors, with easy-to-follow recipes that consider everything from calorie counts to chewability, ensuring that each meal is as enjoyable to eat as it is beneficial for your arthritis. Whether you're cooking for one or a whole family of different ages, these recipes are designed to be shared and enjoyed by all. Each section of this book—from hearty breakfasts to nourishing dinners—is packed with recipes that use simple, wholesome ingredients known for their anti-inflammatory properties. Think vibrant turmeric, zesty ginger, fresh fish, and loads of greens. And we haven't forgotten about dessert; sweet treats can be healthy, too!

Moreover, this cookbook isn't just a collection of recipes; it's a source of support. It includes tips on how to modify your cooking techniques to make kitchen time easier on your joints, advice on how to shop effectively to reduce strain during grocery runs, and strategies to make meal preparation a pleasure, not a pain. The journey with arthritis is as much about mindset as it is about medication. It's about making proactive choices each day that enhance your well-being and maintain your independence. With the "Arthritis Diet Cookbook for Seniors," you hold not just a book, but a tool—a tool that invites you to transform your diet and, by extension, your life.

So, let's begin this culinary journey together. Turn the page, pick out a recipe, and let's start cooking towards a life where arthritis doesn't define your days. Your adventure into delicious, arthritis-friendly cooking starts now.

Chapter 1

Understanding Arthritis in Seniors

The Impact of Arthritis on Daily Life

Arthritis is more than just a medical condition; it's a constant companion that often dictates the pace and quality of one's daily life. For seniors, the presence of arthritis can be particularly challenging, weaving itself into every aspect of their day and transforming even the simplest tasks into hurdles that require courage, patience, and resilience.

Physical Challenges: The Battle Within

Imagine waking up each morning with the hope of a fresh start, only to be met by the persistent ache of stiff joints. For many seniors with arthritis, this is a familiar scenario. The stiffness that greets them at dawn can make the simple act of getting out of bed feel like climbing a mountain. Every movement can become a calculated effort. The once-effortless act of brushing teeth or combing hair might require intricate maneuvering and result in a throbbing reminder of the condition. Walking down the stairs, holding a coffee cup, or even opening a jar can transform into daunting tasks, shrouded in pain and requiring assistance. As the day progresses, so does the toll of arthritis. The burden of physical pain can lead to fatigue, draining the energy needed to engage in daily activities. For some, the act of gardening, playing with grandchildren, or taking a leisurely walk can become rare luxuries instead of everyday joys. The weight of arthritis presses down, making each step a testament to perseverance and endurance.

Emotional Strain: The Silent Struggle

The impact of arthritis is not confined to the body alone. It often carves deep grooves in one's emotional well-being. Seniors, who once reveled in their independence and zest for life, might find themselves feeling frustrated and demoralized. The constant battle with pain and the limitations imposed by arthritis can lead to a sense of loss—loss of independence, loss of mobility, and, at times, loss of identity. Loneliness can become an unwelcome companion. Social activities that were once eagerly anticipated may now seem daunting or out of reach. The fear of pain or the inability to participate fully can lead to isolation, making the world feel smaller and more confined. It's not just about the physical absence from these activities; it's about missing the laughter, the connection, and the sense of belonging that come with them. This emotional toll can also spill over into relationships. Loved ones might struggle to understand the depth of the daily struggle, leading to feelings of guilt or inadequacy for the person with arthritis. They may withdraw, not wanting to burden others with their challenges, which only deepens the sense of isolation.

Adaptation and Resilience: The Path Forward
Despite these formidable challenges, many seniors exhibit remarkable resilience. They learn to adapt, finding new ways to navigate their world and maintain their independence. Assistive devices and home modifications become allies in this journey. Ergonomic utensils, supportive shoes, and grab bars in bathrooms can make a world of difference, offering a semblance of normalcy and ease. Adapting also means making peace with a slower pace. Seniors may find joy in savoring the small moments—listening to a favorite song, reading a cherished book, or enjoying a quiet moment in the garden. These adjustments reflect a profound strength and an unyielding spirit that refuses to be defined by arthritis. Family and friends play a crucial role in this journey. Their understanding, patience, and support can be a lifeline. Simple acts of kindness, like helping with chores or just being present, can lighten the load and bring comfort. For seniors with arthritis, knowing they are not alone in their struggle makes a world of difference.

Common Types of Arthritis in Seniors

Osteoarthritis (OA): The Wear-and-Tear Arthritis

Osteoarthritis, often referred to as the "wear-and-tear" arthritis, is the most common form of arthritis among seniors. It typically manifests as a result of the aging process, where the cartilage—the smooth, protective layer that cushions the ends of bones—gradually deteriorates. This degeneration leads to bones rubbing against each other, causing pain, stiffness, and swelling.

- Symptoms: The primary symptoms of osteoarthritis include joint pain and stiffness, especially after periods of inactivity or overuse. Affected joints may swell, and there might be a loss of flexibility. As the condition progresses, one might hear or feel a grating sensation when using the joint.
- Commonly Affected Joints: Osteoarthritis most commonly affects weight-bearing joints such as the knees, hips, and spine. However, it can also impact the hands, neck, and smaller joints.
- Management: While osteoarthritis is a chronic condition, its symptoms can be managed through a combination of lifestyle changes, physical therapy, medications, and in some cases, surgery. Maintaining a healthy weight, staying active with low-impact exercises, and using supportive devices can significantly alleviate symptoms.

Rheumatoid Arthritis (RA): The Autoimmune Attack

Rheumatoid arthritis is an autoimmune disorder, where the immune system mistakenly attacks the synovium—the lining of the membranes that surround the joints. This leads to inflammation, swelling, and eventually, joint damage.

- Symptoms: RA is characterized by symmetrical joint pain and swelling, meaning it typically affects the same joints on both sides of the body. Common symptoms include joint tenderness, warmth, and stiffness, particularly in the mornings or after periods of inactivity. Fatigue, fever, and weight loss are also common.
- Commonly Affected Joints: RA often begins in smaller joints like those in the hands and feet, but as it progresses, it can spread to wrists, elbows, knees, ankles, and hips.
- Management: Managing RA often requires a comprehensive approach that includes medications to reduce inflammation and prevent joint damage, physical therapy to maintain mobility, and lifestyle adjustments. Early diagnosis and treatment are crucial to slowing the progression of the disease.

Gout: The Sudden Attacker

Gout is a form of arthritis that occurs when uric acid crystals accumulate in the joints, causing sudden and severe episodes of pain, swelling, and redness. It is often linked to dietary factors and can flare up suddenly, often at night.

- Symptoms: Gout attacks are typically acute, with intense pain and swelling, most commonly affecting the big toe, but they can also occur in the ankles, knees, elbows, wrists, and fingers. The affected joint may become extremely tender, warm, and red, making even the lightest touch unbearable.
- Commonly Affected Joints: The big toe is the classic site for gout attacks, but other joints can be involved as well.
- Management: Gout is usually managed with medications that reduce uric acid levels and prevent flare-ups. Dietary changes, such as reducing intake of purine-rich foods (like red meat and alcohol), and maintaining a healthy weight are also critical in managing gout.

Psoriatic Arthritis (PsA): The Dual Struggle

Psoriatic arthritis is an inflammatory type of arthritis associated with psoriasis, a skin condition characterized by red, scaly patches. PsA can affect any joint and often includes symptoms that are similar to both rheumatoid arthritis and osteoarthritis.

- Symptoms: The symptoms of PsA can vary widely. Common signs include joint pain, stiffness, and swelling, often in conjunction with the skin lesions of psoriasis. It can also cause changes in the nails, such as pitting or separation from the nail bed. Enthesitis, inflammation where tendons and ligaments attach to bones, is another hallmark symptom.
- Commonly Affected Joints: PsA can impact any joint in the body, including the spine (leading to spondylitis) and the fingers (causing dactylitis or "sausage fingers").
- Management: Treatment for PsA often involves medications to reduce inflammation and pain, as well as to manage the skin symptoms of psoriasis. Physical therapy and regular exercise can help maintain joint function and mobility.

Ankylosing Spondylitis (AS): The Spinal Invader

Ankylosing spondylitis is a type of inflammatory arthritis that primarily affects the spine, causing chronic pain and stiffness. Over time, it can lead to the fusion of the vertebrae, resulting in a loss of flexibility and a forward-stooped posture.

- Symptoms: Early symptoms often include pain and stiffness in the lower back and hips, especially in the morning or after periods of inactivity. As AS progresses, the pain and stiffness can extend up the spine and into the neck.
- Commonly Affected Joints: The spine is the primary target of AS, but it can also affect other areas such as the shoulders, hips, and even the ribs, making deep breathing painful.

- Management: Managing AS involves a combination of medication to reduce inflammation and pain, and physical therapy to maintain spinal flexibility and posture. Regular exercise, especially activities that promote spinal extension, like swimming or yoga, can be beneficial. In severe cases, surgery may be necessary to correct spinal deformities.

Navigating Life with Arthritis: More Than Just Joint Pain

Living with arthritis means facing a spectrum of symptoms that can vary in intensity and impact from day to day. For seniors, this journey can be particularly challenging as it intertwines with the natural aging process. Here's a closer look at how these common types of arthritis influence daily life and what can be done to manage them:

Osteoarthritis: Coping with Wear-and-Tear

Osteoarthritis (OA) often creeps in slowly, like a shadow growing longer with the setting sun. It's the most familiar form of arthritis for many seniors. The wear-and-tear on the joints over the years takes its toll, making each step or movement a potential source of discomfort.

- Daily Life Impact: The pain and stiffness of OA can make routine activities, like climbing stairs or bending to pick something up, feel daunting. The sense of loss of independence can be profound, affecting not just mobility but also the ability to engage in hobbies or socialize.
- Coping Strategies: Staying active is crucial, despite the pain. Low-impact exercises such as walking, swimming, or gentle yoga can help keep the joints flexible and reduce stiffness. Weight management is also key, as extra weight puts additional stress on already burdened joints.

Rheumatoid Arthritis: The Battle with the Immune System

Rheumatoid arthritis (RA) brings a different kind of struggle, one that is often unpredictable and more intense. The immune system's attack on the joints can lead to severe inflammation and pain that can flare up without warning.

- Daily Life Impact: RA's unpredictable nature can be distressing. Flare-ups can turn a good day into a painful one quickly, affecting the ability to perform simple tasks like buttoning a shirt or opening a door. The fatigue associated with RA can be overwhelming, making even restful activities feel exhausting.
- Coping Strategies: Early and aggressive treatment with disease-modifying medications can help control the symptoms and slow the disease's progression. Incorporating gentle exercises, like stretching or tai chi, can improve joint function. Emotional support from family, friends, or support groups can also play a crucial role in coping with the emotional strain of RA.

Gout: Managing the Sudden Strikes

Gout's sudden and severe attacks can be particularly jarring. The excruciating pain often strikes in the middle of the night, leaving the affected joint swollen and red, and the individual unable to move without intense discomfort.

- Daily Life Impact: Gout can make wearing shoes or walking unbearable during an attack. The fear of a sudden flare-up can make socializing or planning activities difficult, as the pain can significantly limit mobility.
- Coping Strategies: Managing diet and lifestyle is vital for controlling gout. Reducing intake of high-purine foods, staying well-hydrated, and maintaining a healthy weight can help prevent flare-ups. Medications to lower uric acid levels are also essential in managing the condition long-term.

Psoriatic Arthritis: Balancing Skin and Joint Health

Psoriatic arthritis (PsA) adds the complexity of managing both joint and skin symptoms. The pain and stiffness in the joints can be accompanied by the discomfort of psoriasis, making daily life a delicate balancing act.

- Daily Life Impact: PsA can affect multiple joints and cause significant discomfort and disability. The visible nature of psoriasis can also lead to self-consciousness or anxiety about appearance, compounding the challenges of managing the condition.
- Coping Strategies: Treatments for PsA often involve both systemic medications to reduce inflammation and topical treatments for the skin. Regular, gentle exercise can help keep the joints flexible and reduce stiffness. Stress management techniques, like mindfulness or meditation, can be particularly beneficial as stress can exacerbate both psoriasis and PsA symptoms.

Ankylosing Spondylitis: Maintaining Mobility

Ankylosing spondylitis (AS) often strikes in the prime of life but continues into senior years, leading to chronic pain and stiffness primarily in the spine. Over time, it can cause the spine to fuse, severely limiting mobility and posture.

- Daily Life Impact: AS can make daily activities like bending, reaching, or even sitting for long periods painful. As the spine loses its flexibility, maintaining an upright posture can become difficult, impacting not just physical but also psychological well-being.
- Coping Strategies: Regular physical therapy and exercises that focus on maintaining spinal flexibility and good posture are crucial. Pain management strategies, including medications and heat/cold therapies, can provide relief. Staying active and avoiding prolonged periods of inactivity can help prevent further stiffness and loss of mobility.

Symptoms and Diagnosis of Arthritis in Seniors

Recognizing Symptoms: The Body's Early Warning Signs

Arthritis symptoms can range from mild discomfort to debilitating pain, impacting daily life in numerous ways. Recognizing these symptoms early is essential for seeking timely medical intervention. Here's a closer look at the common symptoms associated with arthritis:

Common Symptoms Across Arthritis Types

1. Joint Pain: This is the hallmark of arthritis. Pain can be sharp or dull, constant or intermittent, and can vary in intensity. It often worsens with activity and improves with rest, but for some types of arthritis, the pain can persist even at rest or during the night.
2. Stiffness: Joint stiffness is particularly noticeable in the mornings or after periods of inactivity. Seniors might find it difficult to move their joints or experience a feeling of 'tightness' that eases after some movement.
3. Swelling: Inflammation in the joints often leads to swelling. The affected joint may appear larger than normal, feel warm to the touch, and be tender or painful.
4. Reduced Range of Motion: Arthritis can limit the normal movement of joints. Seniors may find it hard to perform routine activities like bending, reaching, or even walking.
5. Fatigue: Chronic pain and inflammation can lead to significant fatigue, making it hard to carry out daily tasks and reducing overall energy levels.
6. Tenderness: The joints may be tender to the touch, making even light pressure or touch uncomfortable.
7. Visible Redness: In some types of arthritis, the skin over the affected joint may become red and irritated, indicating inflammation.

Specific Symptoms by Arthritis Type

1. Osteoarthritis (OA):
   - Localized Pain: Pain is typically localized to the affected joint(s), such as the knees, hips, or hands.
   - Bony Enlargements: Hard bony lumps may form around the joints.
   - Grinding Sensation: A grating or grinding sensation when moving the joint, known as crepitus, due to the roughening of the cartilage.

2. Rheumatoid Arthritis (RA):

- Symmetrical Symptoms: RA often affects joints symmetrically (e.g., both wrists or both knees).
- Systemic Symptoms: Beyond joint pain, RA can cause systemic symptoms like low-grade fever, loss of appetite, and general malaise.
- Nodules: Firm lumps under the skin near affected joints, known as rheumatoid nodules.

3. Gout:

- Sudden Onset: Gout attacks often begin suddenly, frequently at night, with intense joint pain.
- Red, Warm Joints: The affected joint becomes extremely red, warm, and swollen.
- Tophi: In chronic cases, deposits of uric acid crystals, called tophi, can form under the skin around joints.

4. Psoriatic Arthritis (PsA):

- Skin Symptoms: Presence of red, scaly patches of psoriasis along with joint pain.
- Nail Changes: Pitting or separation of nails from the nail bed.
- Enthesitis: Inflammation where tendons and ligaments attach to the bones.

5. Ankylosing Spondylitis (AS):

- Lower Back Pain: Persistent pain and stiffness in the lower back and hips, particularly in the morning.
- Postural Changes: Gradual stiffening and curving of the spine leading to a stooped posture.
- Reduced Chest Expansion: Limited ability to expand the chest fully, due to involvement of the ribs.

Diagnostic Process: Uncovering the Nature of Arthritis

Diagnosing arthritis involves a comprehensive approach that includes medical history, physical examination, laboratory tests, and imaging studies. Here's how healthcare providers typically go about diagnosing arthritis in seniors:

Medical History

A detailed medical history is the first step in diagnosing arthritis. Physicians will inquire about the onset, duration, and nature of the symptoms, as well as any family history of arthritis or related conditions. They will also ask about the patient's overall health, lifestyle, and any previous injuries or illnesses that might contribute to joint problems.

- Symptom Description: Details about the specific joints involved, the type of pain experienced, and any factors that worsen or relieve the symptoms.
- Family History: Information about any relatives with arthritis or autoimmune diseases.
- Medical and Lifestyle Factors: Discussion about past illnesses, current medications, physical activity level, and dietary habits.

Physical Examination

During the physical examination, the doctor will inspect the affected joints for signs of swelling, redness, and warmth. They will also assess the range of motion, check for tenderness or deformities, and listen for crepitus.

- Joint Inspection: Visual examination and palpation of the joints to detect abnormalities.
- Range of Motion Tests: Evaluating how well the joints move in various directions.
- Symmetry and Deformity Checks: Looking for asymmetry between the left and right sides of the body and checking for joint deformities or nodules.

Laboratory Tests

Lab tests can provide valuable information to support the diagnosis of arthritis and rule out other conditions. Common tests include:

- Blood Tests:
  - Erythrocyte Sedimentation Rate (ESR): Measures inflammation levels in the body.
  - C-Reactive Protein (CRP): Another marker of inflammation.
  - Rheumatoid Factor (RF): An antibody often present in the blood of people with rheumatoid arthritis.
  - Anti-Cyclic Citrullinated Peptide (anti-CCP): A more specific test for rheumatoid arthritis.
  - Uric Acid Levels: High levels can indicate gout.
- Joint Fluid Analysis: Extracting and analyzing fluid from a swollen joint to check for signs of infection, crystals, or other abnormalities.

Imaging Studies

Imaging techniques are crucial for visualizing the internal structures of the joints and assessing the extent of joint damage. Common imaging studies include:

- X-rays: Useful for detecting bone damage, cartilage loss, and the presence of bone spurs in osteoarthritis.
- Magnetic Resonance Imaging (MRI): Provides detailed images of soft tissues, including cartilage, tendons, and ligaments, which is helpful in diagnosing conditions like RA and PsA.
- Ultrasound: Can detect inflammation and fluid accumulation in joints and soft tissues.
- Dual-energy X-ray Absorptiometry (DEXA) Scan: Measures bone density and is particularly useful in diagnosing osteoporosis, which can be associated with arthritis.

Understanding and Managing the Diagnosis

Receiving a diagnosis of arthritis can be overwhelming, especially for seniors. It's not just about understanding the medical terms and treatment plans; it's about coming to terms with a condition that will influence daily life. Here are some steps to help manage the diagnosis effectively:

Building a Support System

Having a network of supportive family, friends, and healthcare providers can make a significant difference. Regular appointments with a rheumatologist, physical therapist, and possibly a dietitian can provide comprehensive care and support.

- Family and Friends: Sharing the diagnosis with loved ones and seeking their support can alleviate feelings of isolation and provide practical help with daily tasks.
- Healthcare Team: Collaborating with a team of specialists ensures that all aspects of the condition are managed, from pain relief to maintaining mobility and function.

Educating Oneself

Knowledge is empowering. Learning about the specific type of arthritis and understanding its symptoms, progression, and treatment options can help seniors make informed decisions about their care.

- Arthritis Education: Attending workshops, reading reputable sources, and joining support groups can provide valuable insights and coping strategies.
- Treatment Options: Understanding the various medications, therapies, and lifestyle changes that can manage arthritis helps in making proactive choices.

Adopting a Positive Outlook

While arthritis can impose significant challenges, maintaining a positive attitude and focusing on what can be controlled is crucial. Engaging in activities that bring joy, practicing mindfulness, and setting realistic goals can enhance quality of life.

- Mindfulness and Stress Management: Techniques like meditation, deep breathing, and yoga can reduce stress and improve mental well-being.
- Staying Active: Regular, gentle physical activity tailored to individual capabilities can help maintain joint function and reduce symptoms.

Chapter 2

The Role of Diet in Managing Arthritis

How Food Affects Inflammation

Inflammation is the body's natural response to injury or infection, a defense mechanism that helps to heal and protect. However, when inflammation becomes chronic, as seen in many types of arthritis, it can lead to persistent pain and damage to the joints. What we eat plays a significant role in either fueling or fighting inflammation in our bodies.

The Science Behind Inflammation and Diet

To appreciate how food influences inflammation, it's essential to understand the biochemical processes involved. Inflammation is driven by the immune system, which releases various chemicals and white blood cells to combat perceived threats. This process is beneficial in short-term scenarios like healing a cut but can be harmful when it becomes chronic.

Certain foods can trigger or exacerbate inflammation, while others possess anti-inflammatory properties that can help calm the body's inflammatory response. The interaction between diet and inflammation involves complex mechanisms, including the production of inflammatory molecules, oxidative stress, and the balance of gut microbiota.

Pro-Inflammatory Foods: Fuelling the Fire

Some foods can contribute to increased inflammation in the body. These are typically rich in substances that promote the production of pro-inflammatory cytokines and oxidative stress, which can aggravate arthritis symptoms.

1. Refined Carbohydrates and Sugars

- Sources: White bread, pastries, candies, sugary drinks, and other processed foods.
- Impact: These foods cause rapid spikes in blood sugar levels, leading to increased production of advanced glycation end products (AGEs), which are known to promote inflammation.

2. Saturated and Trans Fats

- Sources: Red meat, full-fat dairy products, butter, margarine, and processed snacks.
- Impact: Saturated fats can trigger adipose (fat) tissue inflammation, which is linked to arthritis and other chronic conditions. Trans fats, often found in fried and processed foods, are even more harmful and have been directly associated with systemic inflammation.

3. Omega-6 Fatty Acids

- Sources: Vegetable oils (like corn, sunflower, and soybean oil), processed and fried foods.
- Impact: While omega-6 fatty acids are essential in small amounts, excessive consumption can lead to an imbalance with omega-3 fatty acids, promoting inflammation. Modern diets often have a skewed ratio favoring omega-6s, which can exacerbate inflammatory processes.

4. Processed and Red Meats

- Sources: Bacon, sausages, hot dogs, and red meats like beef and pork.
- Impact: These meats contain high levels of saturated fats and AGEs, both of which can trigger inflammation. Additionally, the way these meats are processed and cooked can lead to the formation of inflammatory compounds.

5. Alcohol

- Sources: Beer, wine, spirits, and cocktails.
- Impact: Excessive alcohol consumption can increase inflammation and worsen arthritis symptoms. Alcohol can also interfere with the effectiveness of arthritis medications and damage the liver and other organs.

Anti-Inflammatory Foods: Calming the Flames

On the other side of the spectrum, certain foods have been shown to reduce inflammation and can be powerful allies in managing arthritis. These foods are rich in nutrients, antioxidants, and compounds that can help suppress inflammatory processes and promote overall health.

1. Omega-3 Fatty Acids

- Sources: Fatty fish (like salmon, mackerel, sardines, and trout), flaxseeds, chia seeds, and walnuts.
- Impact: Omega-3 fatty acids are well-known for their potent anti-inflammatory effects. They help reduce the production of inflammatory cytokines and can ease joint pain and stiffness associated with arthritis.

2. Fruits and Vegetables

- Sources: A wide variety of fruits and vegetables, especially leafy greens (like spinach and kale), berries, oranges, and cruciferous vegetables (like broccoli and Brussels sprouts).
- Impact: These foods are rich in antioxidants, vitamins, and fiber. Antioxidants like vitamin C, E, and carotenoids help neutralize free radicals that contribute to inflammation. The high fiber content also promotes a healthy gut microbiome, which plays a crucial role in regulating inflammation.

3. Whole Grains

- Sources: Oats, brown rice, quinoa, barley, and whole-wheat products.
- Impact: Whole grains provide essential nutrients and fiber, which help reduce inflammation. Unlike refined grains, they do not cause rapid spikes in blood sugar and thus help maintain stable glucose levels, which is beneficial in managing inflammatory responses.

4. Nuts and Seeds

- Sources: Almonds, walnuts, flaxseeds, chia seeds, and sunflower seeds.
- Impact: Nuts and seeds are rich in healthy fats, fiber, and antioxidants. They provide anti-inflammatory omega-3 fatty acids and other compounds that can help lower inflammation and protect against chronic diseases.

5. Olive Oil

- Sources: Extra virgin olive oil used in cooking or as a dressing.
- Impact: Olive oil contains oleocanthal, a compound with anti-inflammatory properties similar to non-steroidal anti-inflammatory drugs (NSAIDs). It also provides healthy monounsaturated fats that are beneficial for heart health and inflammation reduction.

6. Herbs and Spices

- Sources: Turmeric, ginger, garlic, cinnamon, and rosemary.
- Impact: Many herbs and spices have strong anti-inflammatory properties. Turmeric, for example, contains curcumin, which has been shown to inhibit inflammatory pathways. Ginger and garlic also contain bioactive compounds that can reduce inflammation and oxidative stress.

7. Legumes

- Sources: Beans, lentils, chickpeas, and peas.
- Impact: Legumes are excellent sources of protein, fiber, and anti-inflammatory phytonutrients. They help stabilize blood sugar levels and provide sustained energy, which is crucial in managing inflammation and overall health.

8. Green Tea

- Sources: Green tea leaves and brewed tea.
- Impact: Green tea is packed with antioxidants, particularly catechins like EGCG (epigallocatechin gallate), which have anti-inflammatory and antioxidant effects. Regular consumption of green tea can help reduce inflammation and support joint health.

9. Berries

- Sources: Blueberries, strawberries, raspberries, and blackberries.
- Impact: Berries are high in vitamins, fiber, and antioxidants like anthocyanins, which help fight inflammation and protect cells from damage. Their anti-inflammatory effects can be beneficial in reducing symptoms of arthritis.

10. Tomatoes

- Sources: Fresh tomatoes, tomato juice, and tomato-based products.
- Impact: Tomatoes are rich in lycopene, an antioxidant with potent anti-inflammatory properties. Cooking tomatoes increases their lycopene content, making them even more effective in reducing inflammation.

Dietary Patterns and Inflammation

Beyond individual foods, overall dietary patterns play a significant role in influencing inflammation. Certain eating patterns are particularly beneficial for managing arthritis and promoting general health.

1. Mediterranean Diet

- Components: Emphasizes fruits, vegetables, whole grains, legumes, nuts, seeds, fish, and olive oil.
- Impact: This diet is known for its anti-inflammatory and heart-healthy properties. It promotes a balance of healthy fats, high fiber, and a variety of nutrients that collectively reduce inflammation and improve joint health.

2. DASH Diet (Dietary Approaches to Stop Hypertension)

- Components: Focuses on fruits, vegetables, whole grains, lean proteins, and low-fat dairy, while limiting sodium, sweets, and red meats.
- Impact: Originally designed to reduce high blood pressure, the DASH diet also helps lower inflammation. Its emphasis on nutrient-dense foods and balanced meals makes it beneficial for managing arthritis.

3. Plant-Based Diets

- Components: Prioritizes plant foods like fruits, vegetables, whole grains, nuts, and legumes, and minimizes or excludes animal products.
- Impact: Plant-based diets are rich in fiber, antioxidants, and anti-inflammatory compounds. They can help reduce inflammation and support overall health, making them a good choice for those with arthritis.

4. Anti-Inflammatory Diet

- Components: Combines elements of the Mediterranean and DASH diets, focusing on anti-inflammatory foods like fatty fish, leafy greens, and berries, while avoiding pro-inflammatory foods.
- Impact: This diet specifically targets reducing inflammation and is tailored to help manage chronic inflammatory conditions like arthritis.

Practical Tips for an Anti-Inflammatory Diet

Adopting an anti-inflammatory diet doesn't have to be difficult or restrictive. Here are some practical tips to help integrate anti-inflammatory foods into your daily routine:

1. Prioritize Fresh, Whole Foods: Focus on incorporating a variety of fresh fruits, vegetables, whole grains, nuts, and seeds into your meals.
2. Choose Healthy Fats: Opt for sources of healthy fats like olive oil, avocados, and fatty fish, and limit intake of saturated and trans fats.
3. Incorporate Herbs and Spices: Use herbs and spices like turmeric, ginger, and garlic to add flavor and anti-inflammatory benefits to your dishes.

4. Limit Sugars and Processed Foods: Reduce consumption of refined sugars and processed foods, which can increase inflammation.

5. Stay Hydrated: Drink plenty of water and include anti-inflammatory beverages like green tea in your diet.

6. Balance Omega-3 and Omega-6 Fatty Acids: Aim for a healthy balance by increasing your intake of omega-3-rich foods and reducing omega-6-heavy foods.

7. Enjoy a Variety of Foods: Eating a diverse range of anti-inflammatory foods ensures you get a wide array of nutrients to support overall health.

8. Mind Portion Sizes: Keep portion sizes in check to maintain a healthy weight, which can help reduce the strain on your joints and decrease inflammation.

9. Plan Ahead: Meal planning and preparation can help ensure you have healthy, anti-inflammatory options readily available, reducing the temptation to reach for less healthy choices.

10. Listen to Your Body: Pay attention to how your body responds to different foods and make adjustments to your diet based on your personal experiences with inflammation and arthritis symptoms.

Nutritional Needs of Seniors with Arthritis

Understanding the Nutritional Challenges

Arthritis can bring several challenges that influence nutritional needs and eating habits among seniors:

1. Reduced Mobility and Pain: Arthritis pain and limited mobility can make it difficult to prepare meals, shop for groceries, or even eat comfortably.
2. Medication Interactions: Certain medications used to manage arthritis can affect appetite, nutrient absorption, or create specific dietary needs.
3. Changes in Metabolism: Aging and reduced physical activity can slow metabolism, requiring adjustments in calorie intake to maintain a healthy weight.
4. Digestive Issues: Some seniors may experience digestive issues, such as slower digestion or difficulty chewing, which can impact nutrient intake.
5. Psychosocial Factors: Loneliness or depression associated with chronic pain can affect appetite and interest in eating.

Essential Nutrients for Seniors with Arthritis

Certain nutrients are particularly beneficial for managing arthritis and supporting overall health in seniors. These nutrients help reduce inflammation, protect joint health, and address common age-related nutritional gaps.

1. Omega-3 Fatty Acids

- Importance: Omega-3 fatty acids are known for their powerful anti-inflammatory properties. They help reduce joint pain and stiffness and support overall joint health.
- Sources: Fatty fish (like salmon, mackerel, and sardines), flaxseeds, chia seeds, walnuts, and omega-3 enriched eggs.
- Recommendations: Aim to include omega-3-rich foods in the diet at least twice a week. Supplements may be considered if dietary intake is insufficient, but it's best to consult with a healthcare provider.

2. Vitamin D

- Importance: Vitamin D plays a crucial role in calcium absorption and bone health. It also has anti-inflammatory effects and may help reduce the risk of autoimmune conditions like rheumatoid arthritis.
- Sources: Sunlight exposure, fortified dairy products, fatty fish, and supplements.
- Recommendations: Seniors should aim for adequate sunlight exposure and consider foods rich in vitamin D or supplements, especially in regions with limited sunlight.

3. Calcium
- Importance: Calcium is essential for maintaining strong bones and preventing osteoporosis, which can be a concern for seniors with arthritis.
- Sources: Dairy products (milk, yogurt, cheese), leafy green vegetables (kale, broccoli), fortified plant-based milks, and calcium supplements.
- Recommendations: Ensure adequate calcium intake through diet and supplements if necessary, especially if there's a risk of bone density loss.

4. Antioxidants
- Importance: Antioxidants help neutralize free radicals that cause inflammation and joint damage. They support overall health and may slow the progression of arthritis.
- Sources: Colorful fruits and vegetables (berries, citrus fruits, leafy greens, bell peppers), nuts, seeds, and green tea.
- Recommendations: Include a variety of antioxidant-rich foods daily to combat oxidative stress and inflammation.

5. Fiber
- Importance: Fiber aids in digestive health, helps control blood sugar levels, and supports a healthy weight, which can reduce the strain on joints.
- Sources: Whole grains, fruits, vegetables, legumes, and nuts.
- Recommendations: Aim for a diet high in fiber by choosing whole foods and incorporating a variety of plant-based sources.

6. Protein
- Importance: Protein is vital for muscle maintenance and repair, which supports joint stability and overall physical strength.
- Sources: Lean meats, poultry, fish, eggs, dairy products, legumes, and plant-based protein sources like tofu and quinoa.
- Recommendations: Include a source of high-quality protein with each meal to support muscle mass and joint health.

7. Magnesium
- Importance: Magnesium is involved in over 300 biochemical reactions in the body, including muscle function and bone health. It helps reduce inflammation and may alleviate arthritis symptoms.
- Sources: Leafy green vegetables, nuts, seeds, whole grains, and legumes.
- Recommendations: Ensure a balanced intake of magnesium through diet, and consider supplements if recommended by a healthcare provider.

8. Vitamin C
- Importance: Vitamin C is crucial for collagen formation, which is essential for healthy joints and cartilage. It also has antioxidant properties that help reduce inflammation.
- Sources: Citrus fruits, strawberries, bell peppers, broccoli, and tomatoes.
- Recommendations: Include vitamin C-rich foods daily to support joint health and reduce inflammation.

9. Zinc and Selenium
- Importance: These trace minerals play a role in immune function and inflammation control. Zinc helps repair tissues, while selenium has antioxidant properties that can help reduce inflammation.
- Sources: Nuts, seeds, whole grains, seafood, and meat.
- Recommendations: Incorporate foods rich in zinc and selenium into the diet to support immune function and manage inflammation.

Foods to Include and Avoid for Seniors with Arthritis

Foods to Include: Anti-Inflammatory Allies
Certain foods possess properties that help fight inflammation, support joint health, and provide essential nutrients needed for overall wellness. Here's a detailed look at foods that should be prioritized in the diet of seniors with arthritis:

1. Fatty Fish
- Examples: Salmon, mackerel, sardines, trout, and anchovies.
- Benefits: These fish are rich in omega-3 fatty acids, which have powerful anti-inflammatory effects. Omega-3s can help reduce joint pain and stiffness, especially in rheumatoid arthritis.
- Serving Suggestion: Aim to include fatty fish in meals at least two to three times a week. Grilled, baked, or broiled preparations are healthier options compared to frying.

2. Colorful Fruits and Vegetables
- Examples: Berries (blueberries, strawberries, raspberries), citrus fruits (oranges, grapefruits), leafy greens (spinach, kale), and cruciferous vegetables (broccoli, Brussels sprouts).
- Benefits: These are packed with antioxidants, vitamins, and minerals that help combat inflammation and oxidative stress. Berries, for instance, contain anthocyanins that reduce inflammation, while greens are rich in vitamin K and calcium, supporting bone health.
- Serving Suggestion: Include a variety of fruits and vegetables in every meal. Fresh, frozen, and even lightly cooked options are beneficial. Aim for a rainbow of colors on your plate to ensure a broad range of nutrients.

3. Whole Grains
- Examples: Oats, quinoa, brown rice, barley, and whole wheat products.
- Benefits: Whole grains are high in fiber, which helps maintain a healthy weight and reduce inflammation. They also provide sustained energy and help control blood sugar levels, which is crucial for overall health and inflammation management.
- Serving Suggestion: Replace refined grains with whole grains in your diet. For instance, choose brown rice over white rice and whole grain bread over white bread.

4. Nuts and Seeds
- Examples: Almonds, walnuts, flaxseeds, chia seeds, and pumpkin seeds.
- Benefits: Nuts and seeds are excellent sources of healthy fats, fiber, and protein. They contain omega-3 fatty acids and antioxidants that reduce inflammation and support heart health.
- Serving Suggestion: Snack on a small handful of nuts or add seeds to salads, cereals, or smoothies. Be mindful of portion sizes as they are calorie-dense.

5. Olive Oil

- Examples: Extra virgin olive oil.
- Benefits: Olive oil is rich in monounsaturated fats and oleocanthal, a compound with anti-inflammatory effects similar to ibuprofen. It's also heart-healthy and supports overall well-being.
- Serving Suggestion: Use olive oil as a primary cooking oil and as a base for salad dressings. Drizzle it over vegetables or use it in marinades.

6. Legumes

- Examples: Beans (black beans, kidney beans), lentils, chickpeas, and peas.
- Benefits: Legumes are high in fiber, protein, and important minerals like iron and magnesium. They help maintain stable blood sugar levels and provide sustained energy while reducing inflammation.
- Serving Suggestion: Include legumes in soups, stews, salads, or as a meat substitute in dishes like chili or tacos.

7. Herbs and Spices

- Examples: Turmeric, ginger, garlic, cinnamon, and rosemary.
- Benefits: Many herbs and spices have potent anti-inflammatory and antioxidant properties. Turmeric's active compound, curcumin, and ginger's gingerol are particularly effective in reducing inflammation and pain.
- Serving Suggestion: Incorporate these spices into cooking or enjoy them as teas. For example, add turmeric to curries, ginger to stir-fries, and garlic to savory dishes.

8. Low-Fat Dairy

- Examples: Low-fat or fat-free yogurt, milk, and cheese.
- Benefits: These provide calcium and vitamin D, essential for bone health. They also offer protein and other nutrients that support overall health.
- Serving Suggestion: Choose low-fat options and incorporate them into meals and snacks. Yogurt with berries, a glass of milk, or cheese with whole grain crackers can be good choices.

9. Green Tea

- Examples: Freshly brewed green tea.
- Benefits: Green tea is rich in catechins, particularly EGCG (epigallocatechin gallate), which have strong anti-inflammatory and antioxidant effects. Regular consumption can help reduce inflammation and protect joints.
- Serving Suggestion: Enjoy green tea hot or cold. Aim for a few cups a day as part of your hydration routine.

10. Tomatoes

- Examples: Fresh tomatoes, tomato juice, and tomato-based products.
- Benefits: Tomatoes are high in lycopene, an antioxidant that helps reduce inflammation. Cooking tomatoes enhances their lycopene content, making them even more beneficial.
- Serving Suggestion: Use tomatoes in salads, soups, sauces, and casseroles. Opt for cooked tomato products like sauces and pastes for a more concentrated dose of lycopene.

Foods to Avoid: Inflammatory Culprits

Certain foods can exacerbate inflammation and should be limited or avoided to help manage arthritis symptoms effectively. These foods are often high in substances that trigger inflammatory responses or contribute to weight gain, which can strain the joints.

1. Refined Carbohydrates and Sugars

- Examples: White bread, pastries, candies, sugary cereals, and sweetened beverages.
- Impact: These foods can cause spikes in blood sugar levels, leading to increased production of pro-inflammatory compounds. They also contribute to weight gain, which puts additional stress on joints.
- Avoidance Tips: Replace refined grains with whole grains and limit sugary snacks and drinks. Opt for natural sweeteners like honey or fruits if you crave something sweet.

2. Saturated and Trans Fats

- Examples: Red meat, full-fat dairy products, fried foods, margarine, and processed snacks.
- Impact: Saturated fats can promote inflammation in fat tissue, while trans fats are even more harmful, directly contributing to systemic inflammation. Both can increase the risk of cardiovascular disease and exacerbate arthritis symptoms.
- Avoidance Tips: Choose lean meats, opt for low-fat dairy, and avoid fried foods and processed snacks. Use healthy fats like olive oil or avocado oil for cooking.

3. Omega-6 Fatty Acids

- Examples: Vegetable oils (corn, sunflower, and soybean oils), processed foods, and certain snack items.
- Impact: While omega-6 fatty acids are essential in small amounts, an excess can lead to an imbalance with omega-3s, promoting inflammation. Modern diets often have an overabundance of omega-6s.
- Avoidance Tips: Balance your intake by increasing omega-3-rich foods and reducing the use of vegetable oils high in omega-6s. Read labels to avoid processed foods with these oils.

4. Processed and Red Meats

- Examples: Bacon, sausages, hot dogs, deli meats, and beef.
- Impact: These meats contain high levels of saturated fats and advanced glycation end products (AGEs), which promote inflammation. They can also contribute to gout and other health issues.
- Avoidance Tips: Limit consumption of red and processed meats. Choose leaner cuts of meat and include more plant-based protein sources like legumes and tofu.

5. Excessive Alcohol

- Examples: Beer, wine, spirits, and cocktails.
- Impact: Excessive alcohol intake can increase inflammation and interfere with the effectiveness of arthritis medications. It can also contribute to weight gain and exacerbate joint pain.
- Avoidance Tips: Limit alcohol consumption to moderate levels, if at all. Consider healthier beverage options like water, herbal teas, or green tea.

6. High-Sodium Foods

- Examples: Processed and canned foods, salty snacks, and restaurant meals.
- Impact: High sodium intake can lead to water retention and increased blood pressure, which may exacerbate joint swelling and inflammation.
- Avoidance Tips: Reduce salt in cooking and choose low-sodium or no-salt-added options. Flavor foods with herbs and spices instead of salt.

7. Artificial Additives

- Examples: Preservatives, colorings, and flavorings found in many processed and packaged foods.
- Impact: Artificial additives can trigger inflammatory responses in some individuals and contribute to overall poor health.
- Avoidance Tips: Opt for fresh, whole foods as much as possible and read labels to avoid products with a long list of artificial ingredients.

Meal Planning and Preparation Tips

Benefits of Meal Planning for Arthritis Management
Meal planning offers numerous benefits, especially for seniors with arthritis. It helps ensure a balanced diet, reduces the stress of daily decision-making, and saves time and energy. Additionally, planning meals can help control portion sizes, manage weight, and ensure the intake of anti-inflammatory foods essential for arthritis management.

1. Consistency in Nutrition: Ensures a steady intake of nutrients essential for managing arthritis.
2. Stress Reduction: Reduces the daily stress of deciding what to eat.
3. Time and Energy Efficiency: Saves time and reduces the physical effort required to prepare meals.
4. Cost-Effective: Helps in budgeting and reducing food waste by planning ahead.
5. Improved Health Outcomes: Supports weight management and overall health, which can alleviate arthritis symptoms.

Key Principles of Meal Planning for Arthritis
Effective meal planning for seniors with arthritis involves several key principles aimed at simplifying the process and maximizing nutritional benefits:

1. Focus on Anti-Inflammatory Foods
- Goal: Incorporate foods that reduce inflammation and support joint health.
- Action: Prioritize fruits, vegetables, whole grains, lean proteins, nuts, seeds, and healthy fats in your meal plans.

2. Balance and Variety
- Goal: Ensure a well-rounded intake of essential nutrients.
- Action: Include a variety of food groups and rotate different foods to avoid monotony and ensure nutritional adequacy.

3. Portion Control
- Goal: Manage weight to reduce stress on joints.
- Action: Plan portion sizes carefully and use measuring tools to avoid overeating.

4. Ease of Preparation
- Goal: Simplify meal preparation to accommodate physical limitations.
- Action: Choose recipes and cooking methods that are easy and require minimal effort or equipment.

5. Incorporate Snacks
- Goal: Maintain energy levels and manage blood sugar.
- Action: Plan for healthy snacks like nuts, fruits, or yogurt to keep energy steady throughout the day.

Practical Meal Planning Strategies
Here are some practical strategies to make meal planning easier and more effective for seniors with arthritis:

1. Create a Weekly Meal Plan
- Steps:
    - Dedicate time each week to plan meals.
    - Consider including a variety of proteins, vegetables, and whole grains.
    - Plan for leftovers to save time on busy days.
    - Use a meal planning template or app to organize your weekly menu.
- Tips:
    - Start with planning a few days at a time if a week feels overwhelming.
    - Incorporate favorite recipes and explore new, easy-to-make dishes.

2. Batch Cooking and Freezing
- Steps:
    - Prepare large quantities of meals and portion them into individual servings.
    - Freeze portions for future use, making sure to label and date them.
- Tips:
    - Choose recipes that freeze well, such as soups, stews, and casseroles.
    - Use freezer-safe containers or bags for easy storage.

3. Pre-Prepare Ingredients
- Steps:
    - Chop vegetables, cook grains, and portion proteins ahead of time.
    - Store prepped ingredients in the fridge for easy access during the week.
- Tips:
    - Invest in ergonomic kitchen tools to make chopping and prepping easier.
    - Consider buying pre-chopped or frozen vegetables to save time and effort.

4. Use Time-Saving Appliances
- Steps:
    - Utilize slow cookers, pressure cookers, and microwaves to simplify cooking.
    - Prepare meals in these appliances to save time and reduce the physical effort required.
- Tips:
    - Look for easy, one-pot recipes that require minimal handling.
    - Set up appliances on a stable surface at a comfortable height to avoid bending or straining.

5. Keep a Stock of Healthy Staples
- Steps:
    - Maintain a well-stocked pantry with essentials like whole grains, canned beans, nuts, seeds, and spices.
    - Ensure the fridge is stocked with fresh fruits, vegetables, and lean proteins.
- Tips:
    - Create a list of staples and keep it handy for regular grocery shopping.
    - Rotate stock to use older items first and avoid waste.

6. Plan for Healthy Snacks
- Steps:
    - Include snacks in your meal plan to maintain energy levels and manage hunger.
    - Choose nutritious options like yogurt, fresh fruit, nuts, or whole-grain crackers.
- Tips:
    - Pre-portion snacks into small containers to grab when needed.
    - Keep snacks accessible and within easy reach to reduce the effort of searching or preparing them.

7. Involve Family or Caregivers
- Steps:
    - Enlist the help of family members or caregivers in meal planning and preparation.
    - Share meal responsibilities, such as shopping, chopping, or cooking.
- Tips:
    - Communicate dietary needs and preferences clearly to those helping.
    - Consider having a family meal prep day to involve everyone and make it a social activity.

Additional Tips for Seniors with Arthritis
1. Use Ergonomic Kitchen Tools: Invest in utensils and gadgets designed to reduce strain on the hands and joints, such as easy-grip knives, jar openers, and lightweight cookware.
2. Organize Your Kitchen: Keep frequently used items within easy reach to minimize bending and stretching. Arrange your kitchen for easy access to ingredients and tools.
3. Take Breaks: Don't feel pressured to complete all meal prep at once. Take breaks as needed to avoid fatigue and joint pain.
4. Stay Hydrated: Drink plenty of water throughout the day. Dehydration can worsen joint pain and fatigue.

5. Listen to Your Body: Pay attention to how your body feels during meal preparation. Adjust tasks or seek help if you experience pain or discomfort.

6. Make Use of Technology: Utilize meal planning apps and online grocery shopping services to simplify the process and save time.

7. Seek Professional Guidance: Consider consulting with a dietitian or nutritionist who can provide tailored advice and support for managing arthritis through diet.

Breakfast Recipes

1. Oatmeal with Berries and Nuts
Ingredients (Serves 2)
- 1 cup old-fashioned rolled oats
- 2 cups water or unsweetened almond milk
- 1/2 cup mixed berries (blueberries, strawberries, raspberries)
- 2 tablespoons chopped almonds
- 1 tablespoon flaxseeds
- 1 tablespoon honey or maple syrup (optional)
- 1/2 teaspoon ground cinnamon

Instructions
1. Prepare Oats: In a medium saucepan, bring the water or almond milk to a boil. Stir in the oats and reduce the heat to low. Cook for about 5 minutes, stirring occasionally, until the oats are tender and have absorbed most of the liquid.
2. Add Cinnamon: Stir in the ground cinnamon and cook for another 1-2 minutes.
3. Serve: Divide the oatmeal into two bowls.
4. Top with Berries and Nuts: Sprinkle the mixed berries, chopped almonds, and flaxseeds evenly over each serving.
5. Drizzle Honey: If desired, drizzle a small amount of honey or maple syrup over the top for added sweetness.

Nutrition Information (Per Serving)
- Calories: 320 kcal
- Protein: 8g
- Carbohydrates: 55g
- Fiber: 9g
- Sugars: 13g (from berries and optional honey)
- Fat: 9g
- Saturated Fat: 1g
- Sodium: 5mg (based on water use)

Cooking Time
- **Preparation Time: 5 minutes**
- **Cooking Time: 10 minutes**
- **Total Time: 15 minutes**

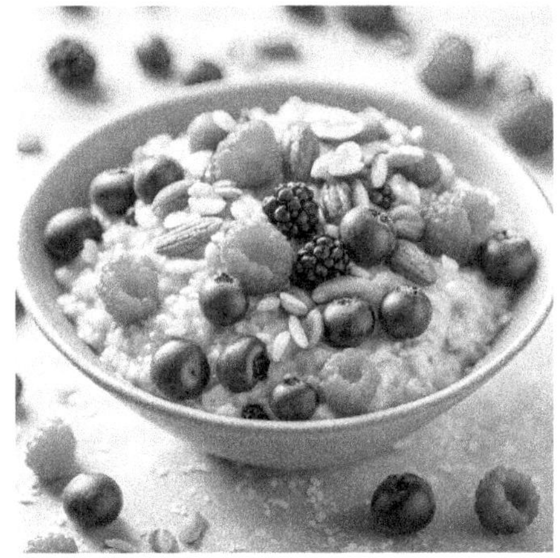

2. Avocado Toast with Cherry Tomatoes

Ingredients (Serves 2)

- 2 slices whole grain or sprouted grain bread
- 1 ripe avocado
- 1/2 cup cherry tomatoes, halved
- 1 tablespoon fresh lemon juice
- 1 tablespoon extra virgin olive oil
- 1 teaspoon red pepper flakes (optional)
- 1/4 teaspoon smoked paprika (optional)
- Fresh basil leaves for garnish (optional)

Instructions

1. Toast Bread: Toast the slices of whole grain bread until golden brown.
2. Prepare Avocado: While the bread is toasting, cut the avocado in half, remove the pit, and scoop the flesh into a bowl. Mash with a fork until smooth. Stir in the lemon juice to add flavor and prevent browning.
3. Spread Avocado: Spread the mashed avocado evenly over the toasted bread slices.
4. Top with Tomatoes: Arrange the cherry tomato halves over the avocado spread.
5. Season and Garnish: Drizzle with extra virgin olive oil and sprinkle with red pepper flakes and smoked paprika, if using. Garnish with fresh basil leaves for added flavor.

Nutrition Information (Per Serving)

- Calories: 290 kcal
- Protein: 5g
- Carbohydrates: 28g
- Fiber: 10g
- Sugars: 3g
- Fat: 20g
- Saturated Fat: 3g
- Sodium: 210mg

Cooking Time

- **Preparation Time: 10 minutes**
- **Cooking Time: 5 minutes**
- **Total Time: 15 minutes**

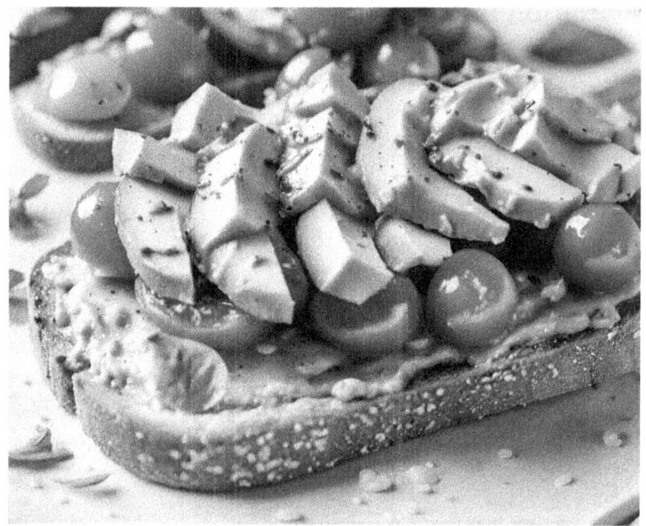

3. Greek Yogurt with Honey and Almonds

Ingredients (Serves 2)

- 1 cup plain Greek yogurt (preferably low-fat or fat-free)
- 2 tablespoons honey
- 2 tablespoons sliced almonds
- 1 teaspoon ground flaxseeds
- 1/4 teaspoon ground cinnamon
- Fresh fruit for topping (optional, such as blueberries or sliced bananas)

Instructions

1. Prepare Yogurt: Divide the Greek yogurt into two bowls.
2. Add Honey: Drizzle 1 tablespoon of honey over each serving of yogurt.
3. Add Almonds and Flaxseeds: Sprinkle 1 tablespoon of sliced almonds and 1/2 teaspoon of ground flaxseeds over each bowl.
4. Season with Cinnamon: Dust with a pinch of ground cinnamon.
5. Optional Topping: Add fresh fruit on top for added flavor and nutrients.

Nutrition Information (Per Serving)

- Calories: 220 kcal
- Protein: 14g
- Carbohydrates: 28g
- Fiber: 2g
- Sugars: 23g (including honey)
- Fat: 7g
- Saturated Fat: 2g
- Sodium: 55mg

Cooking Time

- **Preparation Time: 5 minutes**
- **Cooking Time: 0 minutes**
- **Total Time: 5 minutes**

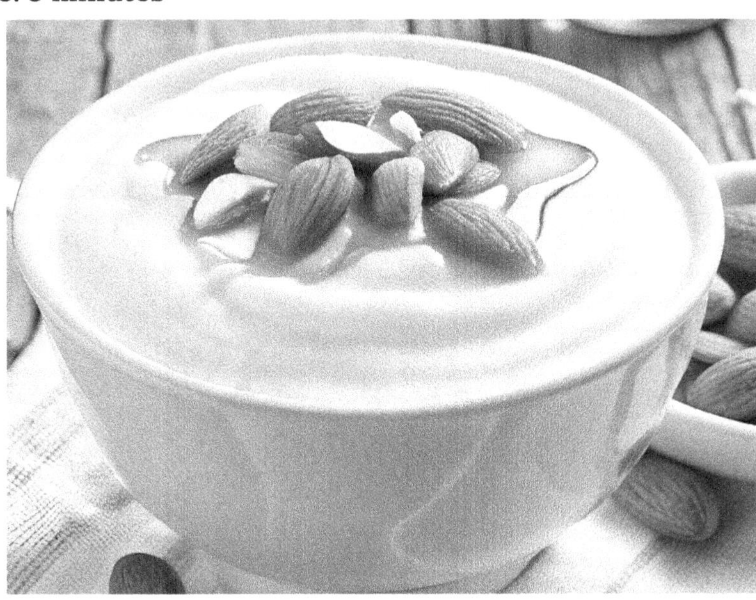

4. Banana and Chia Seed Pudding

Ingredients (Serves 2)

- 1 large ripe banana
- 1 1/2 cups unsweetened almond milk or any preferred plant-based milk
- 1/4 cup chia seeds
- 1 tablespoon pure maple syrup (optional)
- 1 teaspoon vanilla extract
- 1/4 teaspoon ground cinnamon
- Fresh fruit or nuts for topping (optional, such as sliced strawberries or chopped walnuts)

Instructions

1. Blend Banana and Milk: In a blender, combine the banana, almond milk, maple syrup (if using), vanilla extract, and ground cinnamon. Blend until smooth and well combined.
2. Mix in Chia Seeds: Pour the mixture into a medium-sized bowl and stir in the chia seeds. Ensure the seeds are evenly distributed.
3. Refrigerate: Cover the bowl and refrigerate for at least 4 hours or overnight. The chia seeds will absorb the liquid and create a thick, pudding-like consistency.
4. Stir Before Serving: Before serving, give the pudding a good stir to mix the chia seeds evenly throughout the mixture.
5. Top and Serve: Divide the pudding into two bowls. Top with fresh fruit or nuts, if desired, for added texture and flavor.

Nutrition Information (Per Serving)

- Calories: 250 kcal
- Protein: 5g
- Carbohydrates: 40g
- Fiber: 11g
- Sugars: 15g (including natural sugars from the banana)
- Fat: 9g
- Saturated Fat: 1g
- Sodium: 60mg

Cooking Time

- **Preparation Time: 10 minutes**
- **Chilling Time: 4 hours (or overnight)**
- **Total Time: 4 hours 10 minutes**

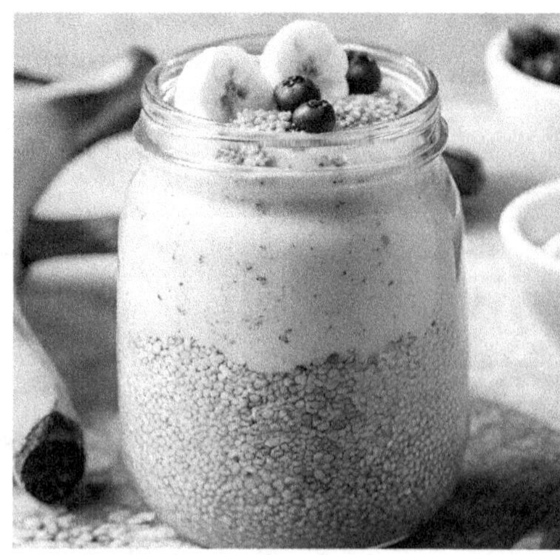

5. Smoothie Bowl with Spinach and Pineapple

Ingredients (Serves 2)

- 2 cups fresh spinach
- 1 cup frozen pineapple chunks
- 1 banana
- 1 cup unsweetened almond milk or coconut water
- 1 tablespoon chia seeds
- 1 teaspoon honey or maple syrup (optional)
- 1/2 cup granola (ensure it's low-sugar and nut-based)
- 1/4 cup fresh berries (blueberries, strawberries)
- 2 tablespoons shredded coconut

Instructions

1. Blend Smoothie: In a blender, combine spinach, pineapple, banana, almond milk (or coconut water), chia seeds, and honey (if using). Blend until smooth and creamy.
2. Serve: Pour the smoothie into two bowls.
3. Top with Toppings: Top each bowl with granola, fresh berries, and shredded coconut.
4. Enjoy: Serve immediately and enjoy a refreshing, nutrient-packed breakfast.

Nutrition Information (Per Serving)

- Calories: 350 kcal
- Protein: 7g
- Carbohydrates: 62g
- Fiber: 10g
- Sugars: 27g (including natural sugars from fruit)
- Fat: 12g
- Saturated Fat: 4g
- Sodium: 50mg

Cooking Time

- **Preparation Time: 10 minutes**
- **Total Time: 10 minutes**

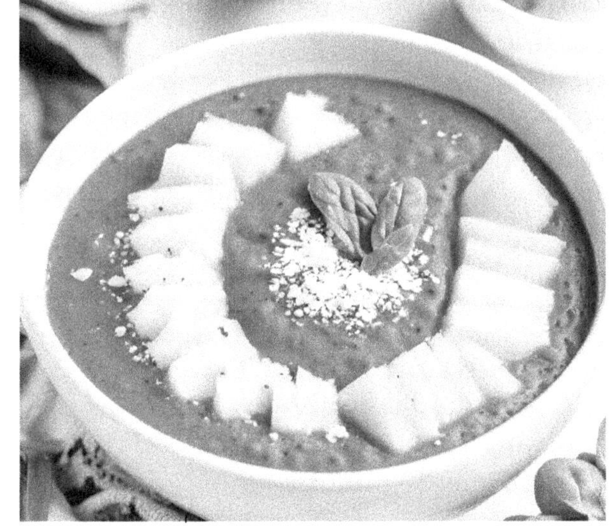

6. Buckwheat Pancakes with Fresh Fruit

Ingredients (Serves 4)

- 1 cup buckwheat flour
- 1 tablespoon ground flaxseed mixed with 3 tablespoons water (flax egg)
- 1 tablespoon baking powder
- 1/2 teaspoon ground cinnamon
- 1 cup unsweetened almond milk
- 2 tablespoons pure maple syrup
- 1 teaspoon vanilla extract
- 1 tablespoon melted coconut oil
- Fresh fruit (like blueberries, strawberries) for topping
- 1/4 cup chopped walnuts (optional)

Instructions

1. Prepare Flax Egg: In a small bowl, combine ground flaxseed with water and let it sit for 5 minutes to thicken.
2. Mix Dry Ingredients: In a large bowl, whisk together buckwheat flour, baking powder, and cinnamon.
3. Combine Wet Ingredients: In another bowl, mix almond milk, maple syrup, vanilla extract, and melted coconut oil. Add the flax egg.
4. Combine: Pour the wet ingredients into the dry ingredients and stir until just combined.
5. Cook Pancakes: Heat a non-stick skillet over medium heat. Pour about 1/4 cup of batter onto the skillet for each pancake. Cook until bubbles form on the surface, then flip and cook until golden brown.
6. Serve: Top pancakes with fresh fruit and walnuts, if desired.

Nutrition Information (Per Serving)

- Calories: 240 kcal
- Protein: 5g
- Carbohydrates: 40g
- Fiber: 6g
- Sugars: 10g (including maple syrup)
- Fat: 8g
- Saturated Fat: 3g
- Sodium: 230mg

Cooking Time

- **Preparation Time: 10 minutes**
- **Cooking Time: 20 minutes**
- **Total Time: 30 minutes**

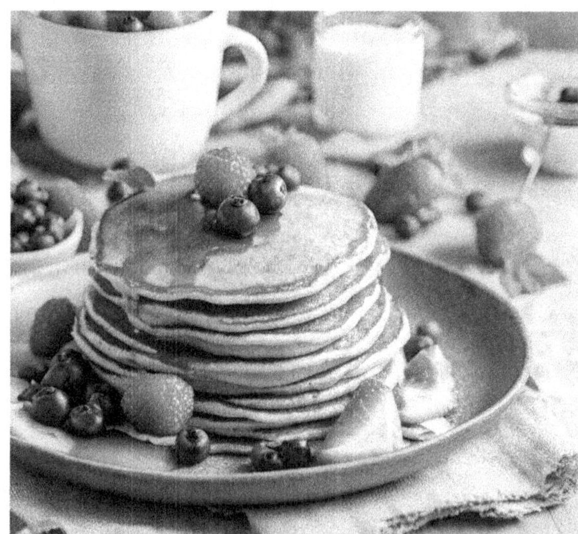

7. Quinoa Breakfast Bowl with Almond Butter

Ingredients (Serves 2)

- 1 cup cooked quinoa
- 1/2 cup unsweetened almond milk
- 1 tablespoon almond butter
- 1 tablespoon honey or agave syrup
- 1/2 teaspoon ground cinnamon
- 1/4 cup mixed berries (blueberries, raspberries)
- 1 tablespoon chia seeds
- 2 tablespoons chopped almonds

Instructions

1. Warm Quinoa: In a small saucepan, combine cooked quinoa and almond milk. Heat over medium-low until warm.
2. Add Flavorings: Stir in almond butter, honey, and cinnamon until well combined.
3. Serve: Divide the quinoa mixture into two bowls.
4. Top with Berries and Nuts: Top each bowl with berries, chia seeds, and chopped almonds.
5. Enjoy: Serve warm for a hearty, nutritious breakfast.

Nutrition Information (Per Serving)

- Calories: 350 kcal
- Protein: 10g
- Carbohydrates: 50g
- Fiber: 10g
- Sugars: 15g (including natural sugars from honey)
- Fat: 14g
- Saturated Fat: 1g
- Sodium: 50mg

Cooking Time

- **Preparation Time: 5 minutes**
- **Cooking Time: 10 minutes**
- **Total Time: 15 minutes**

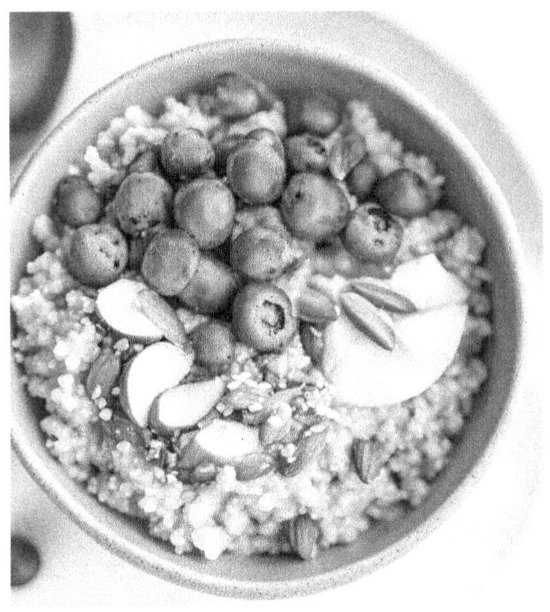

8. Apple and Cinnamon Overnight Oats

Ingredients (Serves 2)

- 1 cup old-fashioned rolled oats
- 1 cup unsweetened almond milk
- 1/2 cup unsweetened applesauce
- 1/2 teaspoon ground cinnamon
- 1/4 teaspoon ground nutmeg
- 1 tablespoon chia seeds
- 1 tablespoon maple syrup (optional)
- 1/2 cup diced apple
- 2 tablespoons chopped walnuts

Instructions

1. Mix Ingredients: In a medium bowl, combine oats, almond milk, applesauce, cinnamon, nutmeg, chia seeds, and maple syrup. Stir until well mixed.
2. Refrigerate Overnight: Divide the mixture into two jars or containers, cover, and refrigerate overnight.
3. Serve: In the morning, stir the oats and top with diced apple and chopped walnuts.
4. Enjoy: Eat directly from the jar or transfer to a bowl.

Nutrition Information (Per Serving)

- Calories: 310 kcal
- Protein: 7g
- Carbohydrates: 50g
- Fiber: 9g
- Sugars: 15g (including natural sugars from apple)
- Fat: 10g
- Saturated Fat: 1g
- Sodium: 45mg

Cooking Time

- **Preparation Time: 10 minutes**
- **Chilling Time: Overnight**
- **Total Time: 10 minutes (plus chilling)**

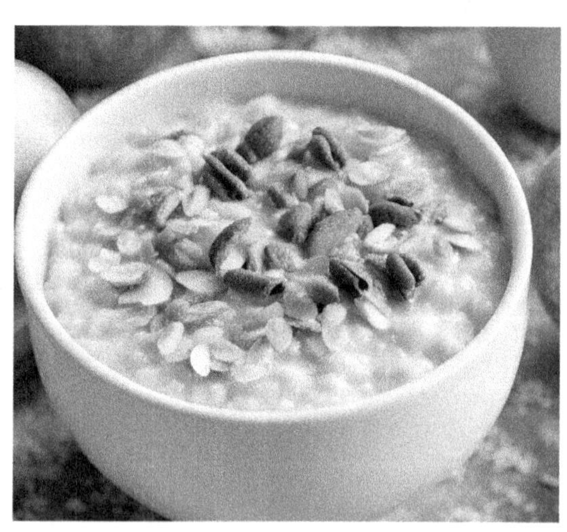

9. Sweet Potato Hash with Kale

Ingredients (Serves 4)

- 2 medium sweet potatoes, peeled and diced
- 1 tablespoon extra virgin olive oil
- 1 teaspoon smoked paprika
- 1 teaspoon ground cumin
- 2 cups chopped kale
- 1/4 cup diced red onion
- 1/4 cup diced bell pepper
- 2 cloves garlic, minced
- Fresh parsley for garnish

Instructions

1. Cook Sweet Potatoes: In a large skillet, heat olive oil over medium heat. Add the sweet potatoes and cook for about 10 minutes, stirring occasionally, until they start to soften.
2. Add Spices: Sprinkle smoked paprika and ground cumin over the sweet potatoes. Stir to coat evenly.
3. Add Vegetables: Add the red onion, bell pepper, and garlic to the skillet. Cook for another 5 minutes, until the vegetables are tender.
4. Add Kale: Stir in the kale and cook until wilted, about 2-3 minutes.
5. Serve: Garnish with fresh parsley and serve warm.

Nutrition Information (Per Serving)

- Calories: 180 kcal
- Protein: 3g
- Carbohydrates: 30g
- Fiber: 6g
- Sugars: 7g
- Fat: 6g
- Saturated Fat: 1g
- Sodium: 60mg

Cooking Time

- **Preparation Time: 10 minutes**
- **Cooking Time: 20 minutes**
- **Total Time: 30 minutes**

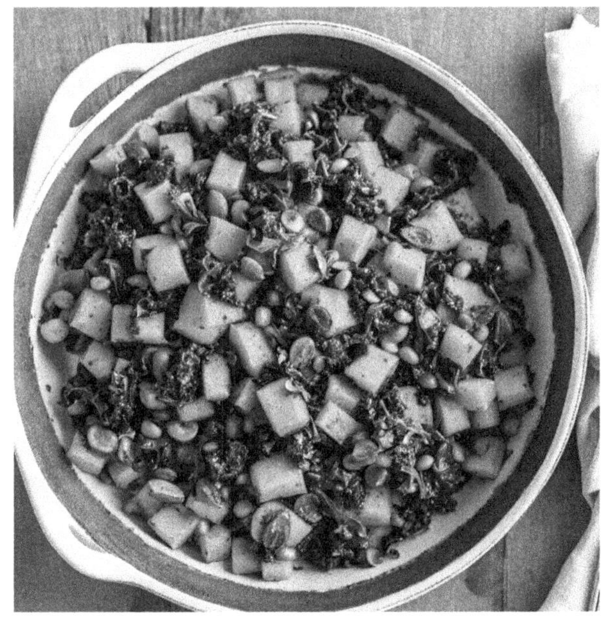

10. Almond Flour Muffins with Blueberries

Ingredients (Serves 12 Muffins)

- 2 cups almond flour
- 1/2 teaspoon baking soda
- 1/4 teaspoon ground cinnamon
- 2 large eggs
- 1/4 cup pure maple syrup
- 1/4 cup unsweetened applesauce
- 1 teaspoon vanilla extract
- 1 cup fresh or frozen blueberries
- 2 tablespoons sliced almonds (optional)

Instructions

1. Preheat Oven: Preheat your oven to 350°F (175°C). Line a muffin tin with paper liners or grease lightly with oil.
2. Mix Dry Ingredients: In a large bowl, whisk together almond flour, baking soda, and cinnamon.
3. Combine Wet Ingredients: In another bowl, beat the eggs, maple syrup, applesauce, and vanilla extract until well blended.
4. Combine and Fold: Add the wet ingredients to the dry ingredients and mix until just combined. Gently fold in the blueberries.
5. Fill Muffin Tin: Spoon the batter into the prepared muffin tin, filling each cup about 3/4 full. Sprinkle with sliced almonds, if using.
6. Bake: Bake for 20-25 minutes, or until a toothpick inserted into the center comes out clean.
7. Cool: Allow the muffins to cool in the tin for 5 minutes before transferring to a wire rack to cool completely.

Nutrition Information (Per Muffin)

- Calories: 160 kcal
- Protein: 5g
- Carbohydrates: 12g
- Fiber: 3g
- Sugars: 8g (including natural sugars from blueberries)
- Fat: 11g
- Saturated Fat: 1g
- Sodium: 70mg

Cooking Time

- **Preparation Time: 10 minutes**
- **Cooking Time: 25 minutes**
- **Total Time: 35 minutes**

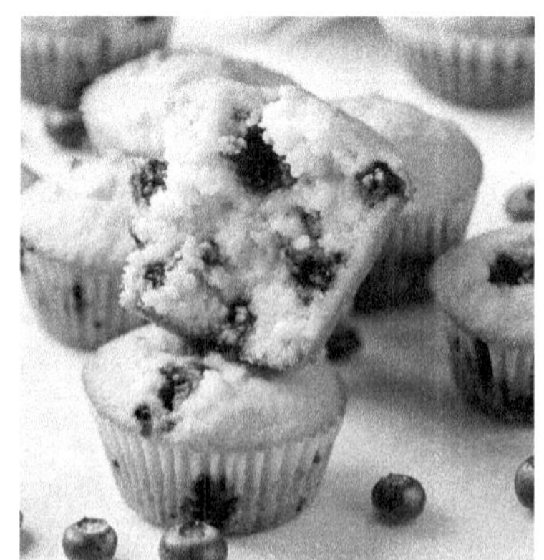

11. Mango and Turmeric Smoothie

Ingredients (Serves 2)

- 1 cup frozen mango chunks
- 1/2 cup fresh orange juice
- 1/2 cup unsweetened coconut milk
- 1/2 teaspoon ground turmeric
- 1/4 teaspoon ground ginger
- 1 tablespoon chia seeds
- 1 teaspoon honey or agave syrup (optional)

Instructions

1. Blend Ingredients: In a blender, combine the mango chunks, orange juice, coconut milk, turmeric, ginger, chia seeds, and honey (if using). Blend until smooth and creamy.
2. Serve: Pour into two glasses and enjoy immediately.

Nutrition Information (Per Serving)

- Calories: 180 kcal
- Protein: 2g
- Carbohydrates: 34g
- Fiber: 5g
- Sugars: 26g (including natural sugars from mango and orange juice)
- Fat: 6g
- Saturated Fat: 4g
- Sodium: 15mg

Cooking Time

- **Preparation Time: 5 minutes**
- **Total Time: 5 minutes**

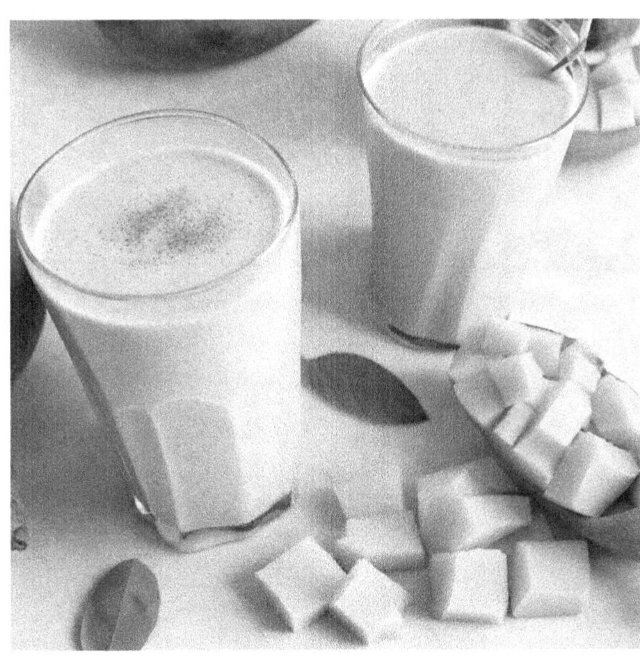

12. Cottage Cheese with Pineapple and Walnuts

Ingredients (Serves 2)

- 1 cup low-fat cottage cheese
- 1/2 cup fresh or canned pineapple chunks (in juice, not syrup)
- 2 tablespoons chopped walnuts
- 1 tablespoon honey or agave syrup (optional)
- 1/4 teaspoon ground cinnamon

Instructions

1. Prepare Cottage Cheese: Divide the cottage cheese into two bowls.
2. Add Pineapple: Top each serving with pineapple chunks.
3. Add Walnuts: Sprinkle chopped walnuts over the pineapple.
4. Drizzle Honey: Drizzle honey over the top if using.
5. Season with Cinnamon: Sprinkle a pinch of ground cinnamon for extra flavor.
6. Serve: Enjoy as a refreshing, protein-packed breakfast or snack.

Nutrition Information (Per Serving)

- Calories: 200 kcal
- Protein: 15g
- Carbohydrates: 18g
- Fiber: 2g
- Sugars: 14g (including natural sugars from pineapple)
- Fat: 8g
- Saturated Fat: 2g
- Sodium: 400mg

Cooking Time

- **Preparation Time: 5 minutes**
- **Total Time: 5 minutes**

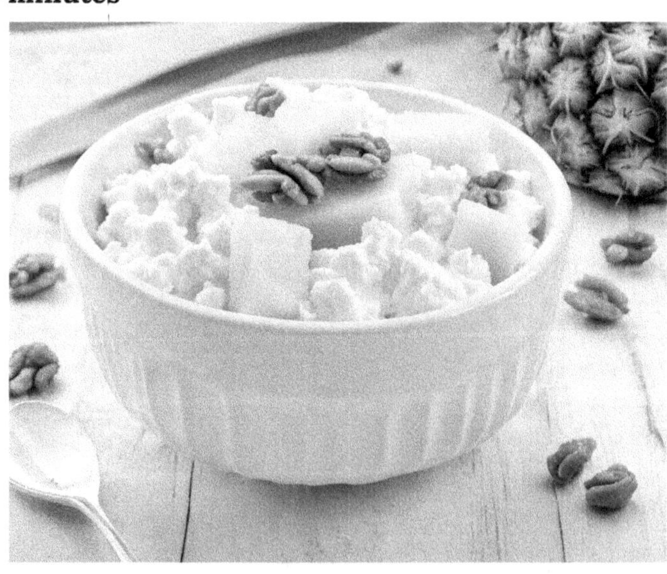

13. Green Tea and Berry Smoothie
Ingredients (Serves 2)
- 1 cup brewed green tea, cooled
- 1 cup frozen mixed berries (blueberries, raspberries, strawberries)
- 1 banana
- 1/2 cup unsweetened almond milk
- 1 tablespoon chia seeds
- 1 tablespoon honey or maple syrup (optional)

Instructions
1. Brew Green Tea: Brew 1 cup of green tea and let it cool to room temperature.
2. Blend Ingredients: In a blender, combine the brewed green tea, frozen berries, banana, almond milk, chia seeds, and honey (if using). Blend until smooth.
3. Serve: Pour into two glasses and enjoy immediately.

Nutrition Information (Per Serving)
- Calories: 160 kcal
- Protein: 3g
- Carbohydrates: 34g
- Fiber: 8g
- Sugars: 17g (including natural sugars from fruit)
- Fat: 3g
- Saturated Fat: 0.5g
- Sodium: 45mg

Cooking Time
- **Preparation Time: 5 minutes**
- **Total Time: 5 minutes**

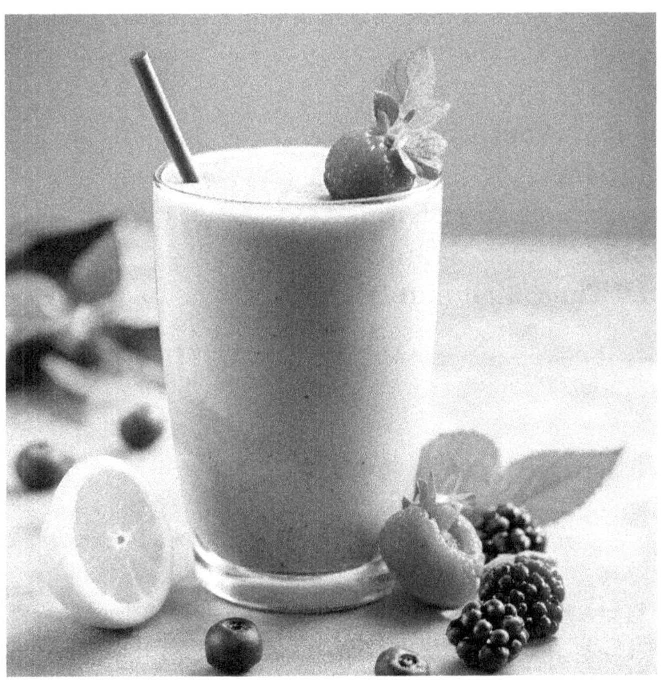

14. Millet Porridge with Almonds and Raisins

Ingredients (Serves 2)

- 1/2 cup millet
- 1 1/2 cups water
- 1/2 cup unsweetened almond milk
- 1/4 cup raisins
- 2 tablespoons chopped almonds
- 1 tablespoon honey or agave syrup (optional)
- 1/2 teaspoon ground cinnamon

Instructions

1. Cook Millet: In a medium saucepan, bring water to a boil. Add millet, reduce heat to low, cover, and simmer for about 15-20 minutes until the millet is tender and the water is absorbed.
2. Add Milk and Mix-ins: Stir in almond milk, raisins, and cinnamon. Continue to cook on low for an additional 5 minutes, stirring occasionally until the mixture is creamy.
3. Serve: Divide the porridge into two bowls. Drizzle with honey, if using, and sprinkle with chopped almonds.
4. Enjoy: Serve warm and enjoy a hearty breakfast.

Nutrition Information (Per Serving)

- Calories: 290 kcal
- Protein: 6g
- Carbohydrates: 48g
- Fiber: 6g
- Sugars: 16g (including natural sugars from raisins)
- Fat: 9g
- Saturated Fat: 1g
- Sodium: 40mg

Cooking Time

- **Preparation Time: 5 minutes**
- **Cooking Time: 25 minutes**
- **Total Time: 30 minutes**

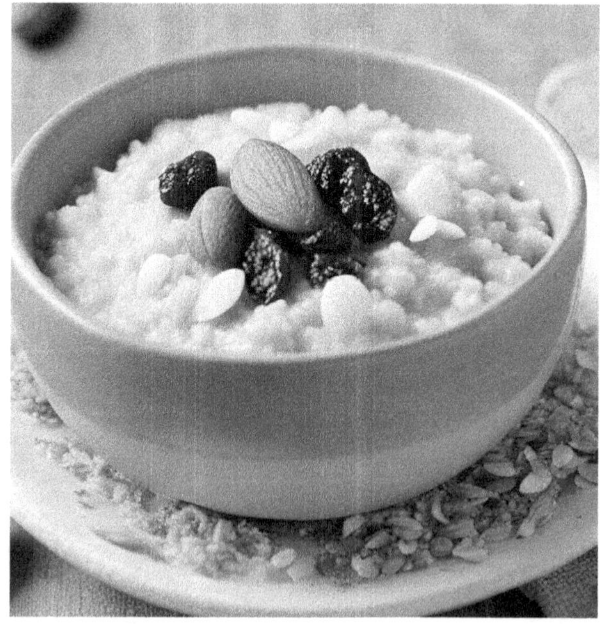

15. Egg White Omelette with Bell Peppers and Onions

Ingredients (Serves 2)

- 6 large egg whites
- 1/4 cup diced red bell pepper
- 1/4 cup diced green bell pepper
- 1/4 cup diced yellow onion
- 1 tablespoon extra virgin olive oil
- 1/4 teaspoon turmeric powder
- Fresh parsley for garnish (optional)

Instructions

1. Prep Vegetables: Heat olive oil in a non-stick skillet over medium heat. Add diced bell peppers and onion. Cook for about 5 minutes until softened.
2. Whisk Egg Whites: In a bowl, whisk the egg whites and turmeric powder until frothy.
3. Cook Omelette: Pour the egg whites into the skillet over the vegetables. Cook for 2-3 minutes, gently lifting the edges to let uncooked egg flow underneath.
4. Fold and Serve: Once set, fold the omelette in half and cook for another minute. Slide onto a plate and garnish with fresh parsley.
5. Enjoy: Serve warm.

Nutrition Information (Per Serving)

- Calories: 120 kcal
- Protein: 12g
- Carbohydrates: 5g
- Fiber: 1g
- Sugars: 2g
- Fat: 6g
- Saturated Fat: 1g
- Sodium: 140mg

Cooking Time

- **Preparation Time: 5 minutes**
- **Cooking Time: 10 minutes**
- **Total Time: 15 minutes**

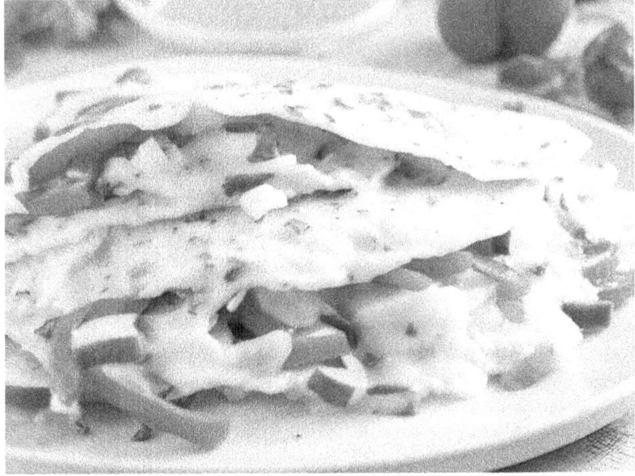

16. Chia and Flaxseed Porridge
Ingredients (Serves 2)

- 1/4 cup chia seeds
- 2 tablespoons ground flaxseeds
- 1 1/2 cups unsweetened almond milk
- 1 tablespoon honey or maple syrup (optional)
- 1 teaspoon vanilla extract
- 1/2 teaspoon ground cinnamon
- Fresh fruit (like sliced banana or berries) for topping

Instructions

1. Mix Ingredients: In a medium bowl, combine chia seeds, ground flaxseeds, almond milk, honey, vanilla extract, and cinnamon. Stir well to combine.
2. Refrigerate: Cover and refrigerate for at least 30 minutes, or overnight, until thickened.
3. Stir and Serve: Stir the porridge to mix well. Divide into two bowls.
4. Add Toppings: Top with fresh fruit and serve chilled or at room temperature.

Nutrition Information (Per Serving)

- Calories: 220 kcal
- Protein: 7g
- Carbohydrates: 23g
- Fiber: 11g
- Sugars: 8g (including natural sugars from fruit)
- Fat: 11g
- Saturated Fat: 1g
- Sodium: 50mg

Cooking Time

- **Preparation Time: 5 minutes**
- **Chilling Time: 30 minutes (or overnight)**
- **Total Time: 35 minutes (including chilling)**

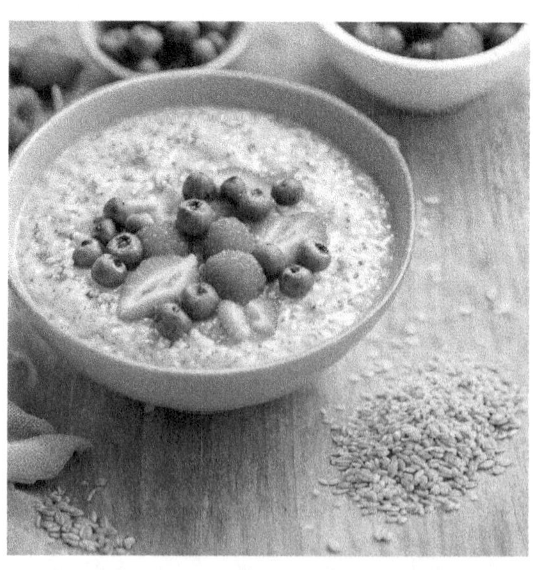

17. Baked Apples with Cinnamon and Walnuts

Ingredients (Serves 2)

- 2 medium apples (Granny Smith or Honeycrisp)
- 2 tablespoons chopped walnuts
- 1 tablespoon pure maple syrup
- 1 teaspoon ground cinnamon
- 1/4 teaspoon ground nutmeg
- 1/4 teaspoon ground ginger

Instructions

1. Preheat Oven: Preheat your oven to 350°F (175°C).
2. Core Apples: Core the apples, leaving the bottom intact to hold the filling.
3. Fill Apples: In a small bowl, mix walnuts, maple syrup, cinnamon, nutmeg, and ginger.
4. Bake Apples: Place the filled apples in a baking dish. Add about 1/4 inch of water to the bottom of the dish to keep the apples moist during baking. Cover with aluminum foil and bake for 25-30 minutes until the apples are tender.
5. Serve: Remove from the oven and let them cool slightly. Serve warm.

Nutrition Information (Per Serving)

- Calories: 180 kcal
- Protein: 2g
- Carbohydrates: 35g
- Fiber: 7g
- Sugars: 24g (natural sugars from apples and maple syrup)
- Fat: 6g
- Saturated Fat: 0.5g
- Sodium: 2mg

Cooking Time

- **Preparation Time: 10 minutes**
- **Cooking Time: 30 minutes**
- **Total Time: 40 minutes**

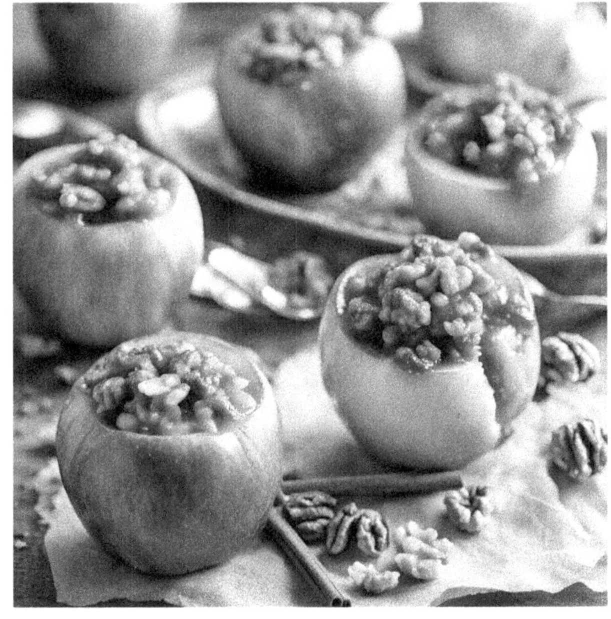

18. Lentil Breakfast Bowl with Spinach

Ingredients (Serves 2)

- 1 cup cooked lentils (brown or green)
- 2 cups fresh spinach
- 1/2 cup cherry tomatoes, halved
- 1/4 cup diced red onion
- 1 tablespoon extra virgin olive oil
- 1 teaspoon turmeric powder
- 1 teaspoon ground cumin
- 1 tablespoon fresh lemon juice
- Fresh parsley for garnish (optional)

Instructions

1. Cook Lentils: If not already cooked, cook the lentils according to the package instructions.
2. Sauté Vegetables: In a medium skillet, heat olive oil over medium heat. Add the diced red onion and cook for 2-3 minutes until translucent. Add the cherry tomatoes and spinach and cook until the spinach is wilted.
3. Combine Lentils and Spices: Add the cooked lentils to the skillet. Sprinkle with turmeric and cumin. Stir to combine and heat through.
4. Finish with Lemon Juice: Remove from heat and stir in the fresh lemon juice.
5. Serve: Divide the mixture into two bowls. Garnish with fresh parsley, if desired, and serve warm.

Nutrition Information (Per Serving)

- Calories: 250 kcal
- Protein: 12g
- Carbohydrates: 32g
- Fiber: 11g
- Sugars: 6g (natural sugars from vegetables)
- Fat: 9g
- Saturated Fat: 1g
- Sodium: 45mg

Cooking Time

- **Preparation Time: 10 minutes**
- **Cooking Time: 10 minutes**
- **Total Time: 20 minutes**

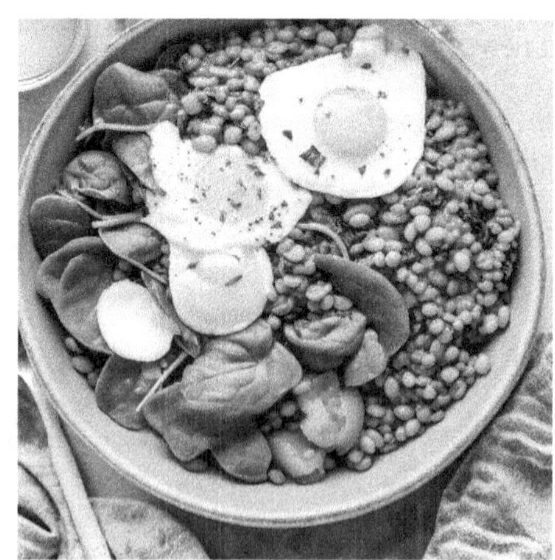

19. Pumpkin and Oat Breakfast Bars

Ingredients (Serves 12 Bars)

- 2 cups rolled oats
- 1 cup canned pumpkin puree (unsweetened)
- 1/2 cup almond butter
- 1/4 cup pure maple syrup
- 1/4 cup unsweetened applesauce
- 1 teaspoon vanilla extract
- 1 teaspoon ground cinnamon
- 1/2 teaspoon ground nutmeg
- 1/4 teaspoon ground ginger
- 1/4 cup chopped walnuts (optional)

Instructions

1. Preheat Oven: Preheat your oven to 350°F (175°C). Line a baking pan with parchment paper.
2. Mix Wet Ingredients: In a large bowl, mix the pumpkin puree, almond butter, maple syrup, applesauce, and vanilla extract until smooth.
3. Add Dry Ingredients: Stir in the oats, cinnamon, nutmeg, ginger, and chopped walnuts (if using) until well combined.
4. Bake Bars: Spread the mixture evenly in the prepared baking pan. Bake for 25-30 minutes until the edges are golden brown.
5. Cool and Cut: Allow the bars to cool completely in the pan. Lift them out using the parchment paper and cut into 12 bars.
6. Serve: Enjoy the bars for breakfast or as a snack.

Nutrition Information (Per Bar)

- Calories: 160 kcal
- Protein: 4g
- Carbohydrates: 20g
- Fiber: 3g
- Sugars: 8g (including natural sugars from maple syrup and applesauce)
- Fat: 7g
- Saturated Fat: 1g
- Sodium: 10mg

Cooking Time

- **Preparation Time: 10 minutes**
- **Cooking Time: 30 minutes**
- **Total Time: 40 minutes**

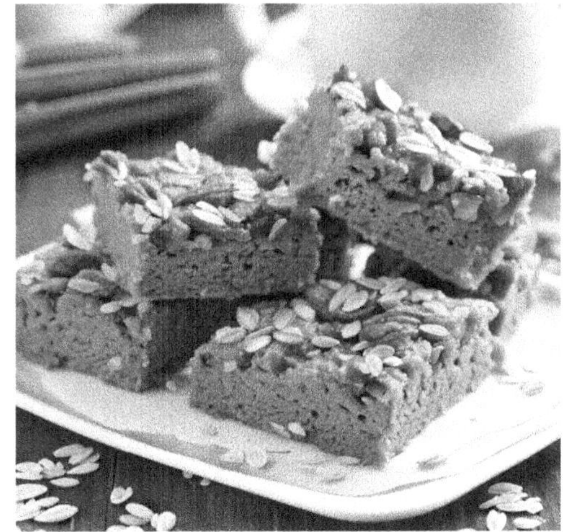

20. Smoked Salmon and Avocado Toast

Ingredients (Serves 2)

- 2 slices whole grain or rye bread
- 1 ripe avocado
- 1/4 teaspoon ground black pepper
- 1 tablespoon fresh lemon juice
- 4 ounces smoked salmon
- 1 tablespoon capers
- Fresh dill for garnish (optional)

Instructions

1. Toast Bread: Toast the slices of whole grain bread until golden and crispy.
2. Prepare Avocado: While the bread is toasting, cut the avocado in half, remove the pit, and scoop the flesh into a bowl. Mash with a fork until smooth. Stir in the lemon juice and ground black pepper.
3. Assemble Toast: Spread the mashed avocado evenly over the toasted bread slices.
4. Add Salmon and Capers: Place slices of smoked salmon on top of the avocado spread. Sprinkle with capers.
5. Garnish and Serve: Garnish with fresh dill if desired. Serve immediately.

Nutrition Information (Per Serving)

- Calories: 300 kcal
- Protein: 14g
- Carbohydrates: 24g
- Fiber: 8g
- Sugars: 2g
- Fat: 18g
- Saturated Fat: 3g
- Sodium: 500mg

Cooking Time

- **Preparation Time: 10 minutes**
- **Total Time: 10 minutes**

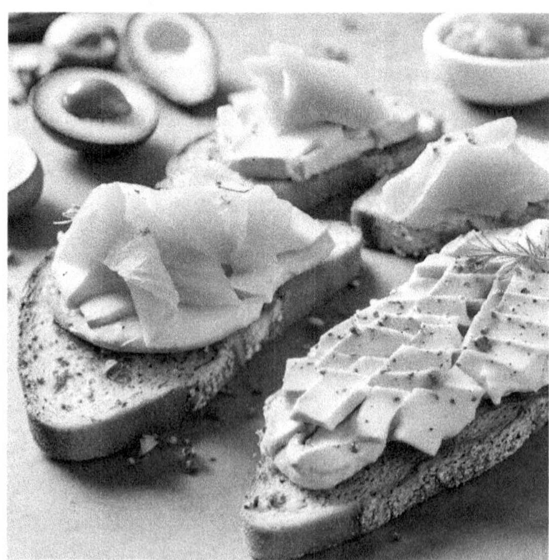

21. Berry and Almond Smoothie

Ingredients (Serves 2)

- 1 cup unsweetened almond milk
- 1 cup mixed frozen berries (blueberries, strawberries, raspberries)
- 1 banana
- 2 tablespoons almond butter
- 1 tablespoon chia seeds
- 1 teaspoon honey or maple syrup (optional)
- 1/2 teaspoon vanilla extract

Instructions

1. Blend Ingredients: In a blender, combine the almond milk, mixed berries, banana, almond butter, chia seeds, honey (if using), and vanilla extract.
2. Blend Smooth: Blend until smooth and creamy.
3. Serve: Pour into two glasses and serve immediately.

Nutrition Information (Per Serving)

- Calories: 250 kcal
- Protein: 6g
- Carbohydrates: 38g
- Fiber: 8g
- Sugars: 20g (including natural sugars from fruit)
- Fat: 10g
- Saturated Fat: 1g
- Sodium: 90mg

Cooking Time

- **Preparation Time: 5 minutes**
- **Total Time: 5 minutes**

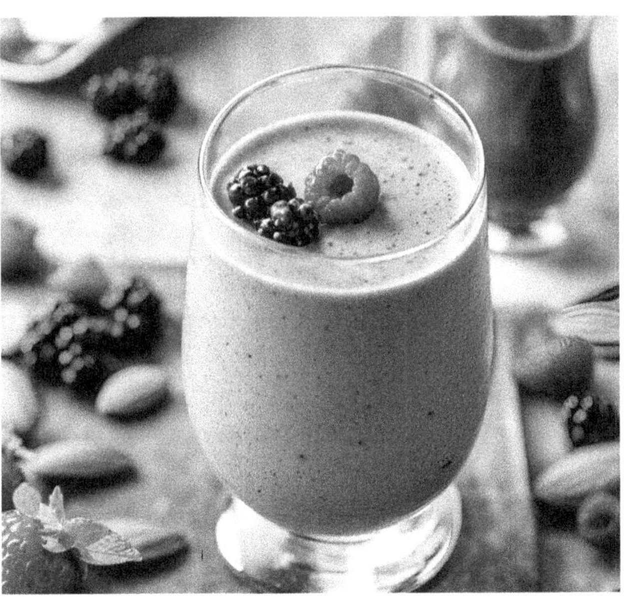

22. Mixed Nut and Fruit Breakfast Bowl

Ingredients (Serves 2)

- 1 cup plain Greek yogurt (preferably low-fat or fat-free)
- 1/2 cup mixed nuts (almonds, walnuts, pistachios)
- 1/2 cup mixed fresh fruit (like berries, apple slices, or banana slices)
- 1 tablespoon chia seeds
- 1 tablespoon flaxseeds
- 1 teaspoon honey or agave syrup (optional)
- 1/2 teaspoon ground cinnamon

Instructions

1. Prepare Yogurt Base: Divide the Greek yogurt into two bowls.
2. Add Toppings: Top each bowl with an even distribution of mixed nuts, fresh fruit, chia seeds, and flaxseeds.
3. Add Sweetener and Cinnamon: Drizzle honey or agave syrup over the top if using, and sprinkle with ground cinnamon.
4. Serve: Enjoy as a nutrient-packed, protein-rich breakfast.

Nutrition Information (Per Serving)

- Calories: 350 kcal
- Protein: 18g
- Carbohydrates: 30g
- Fiber: 8g
- Sugars: 15g (including natural sugars from fruit)
- Fat: 18g
- Saturated Fat: 3g
- Sodium: 100mg

Cooking Time

- **Preparation Time: 5 minutes**
- **Total Time: 5 minutes**

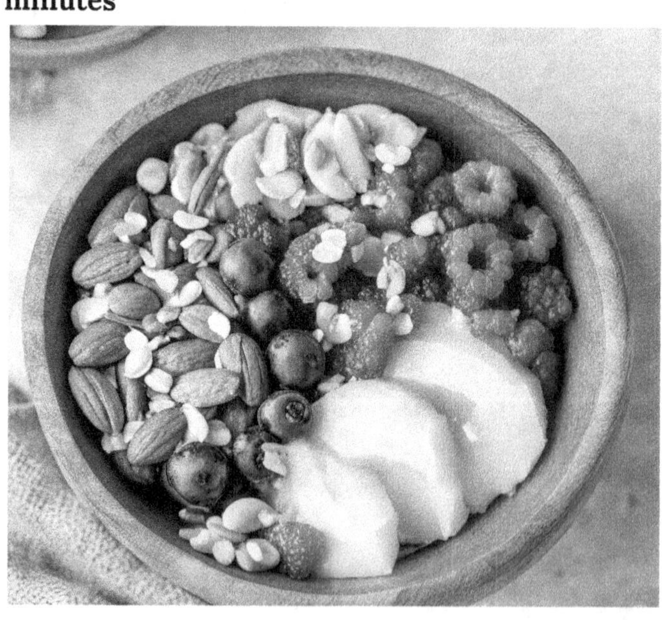

23. Quinoa and Blueberry Breakfast Parfait

Ingredients (Serves 2)

- 1 cup cooked quinoa, cooled
- 1 cup plain Greek yogurt (preferably low-fat or fat-free)
- 1/2 cup fresh blueberries
- 2 tablespoons honey or agave syrup
- 1/4 teaspoon ground cinnamon
- 2 tablespoons chopped walnuts

Instructions

1. Layer Ingredients: In two glasses or bowls, layer 1/4 cup of the cooked quinoa, followed by 1/4 cup of Greek yogurt.
2. Add Blueberries and Honey: Add a layer of fresh blueberries, then drizzle with 1 tablespoon of honey or agave syrup.
3. Repeat Layers: Repeat the layers of quinoa, yogurt, and blueberries.
4. Top with Nuts and Cinnamon: Finish with a sprinkle of chopped walnuts and a pinch of ground cinnamon.
5. Serve: Serve immediately or refrigerate for later enjoyment.

Nutrition Information (Per Serving)

- Calories: 290 kcal
- Protein: 12g
- Carbohydrates: 42g
- Fiber: 5g
- Sugars: 22g (including natural sugars from honey and blueberries)
- Fat: 9g
- Saturated Fat: 2g
- Sodium: 60mg

Cooking Time

- **Preparation Time: 10 minutes**
- **Total Time: 10 minutes**

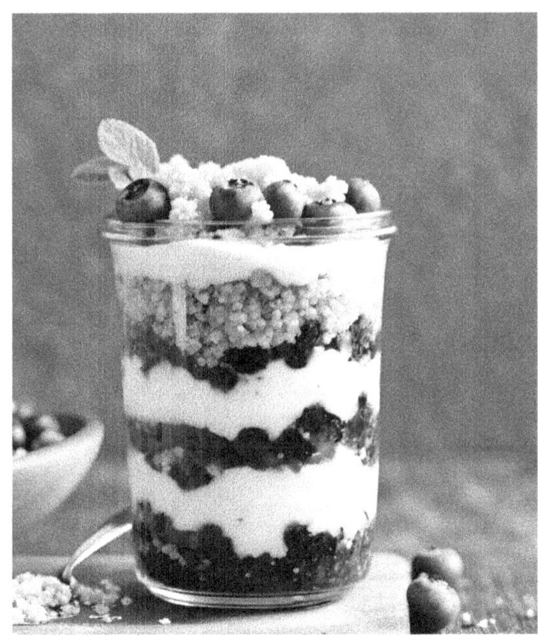

24. Pumpkin Seed and Apple Muesli

Ingredients (Serves 2)

- 1 cup rolled oats
- 1/2 cup unsweetened almond milk
- 1/2 cup unsweetened apple juice
- 1/4 cup grated apple
- 2 tablespoons pumpkin seeds
- 2 tablespoons chopped almonds
- 1 tablespoon honey or maple syrup (optional)
- 1/2 teaspoon ground cinnamon

Instructions

1. Mix Dry Ingredients: In a medium bowl, combine the rolled oats, pumpkin seeds, and chopped almonds.
2. Add Liquid and Fruit: Stir in the almond milk, apple juice, and grated apple. Mix well.
3. Sweeten and Flavor: Add honey or maple syrup if using, and sprinkle with ground cinnamon.
4. Refrigerate: Cover and refrigerate for at least 30 minutes, or overnight, to allow the oats to soften and flavors to meld.
5. Serve: Stir the muesli before serving. Divide into two bowls and enjoy chilled or at room temperature.

Nutrition Information (Per Serving)

- Calories: 280 kcal
- Protein: 8g
- Carbohydrates: 42g
- Fiber: 7g
- Sugars: 18g (including natural sugars from apple and juice)
- Fat: 10g
- Saturated Fat: 1g
- Sodium: 25mg

Cooking Time

- **Preparation Time: 10 minutes**
- **Chilling Time: 30 minutes (or overnight)**
- **Total Time: 40 minutes (including chilling)**

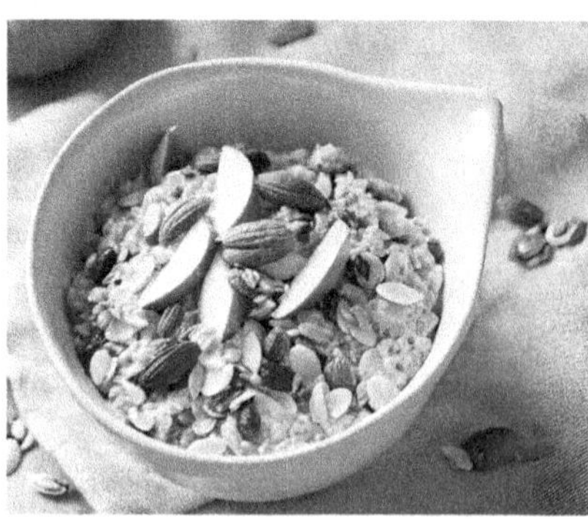

Fish and Seafood Recipes

1. Baked Salmon with Lemon and Dill

Ingredients (Serves 4)

- 4 salmon fillets (about 6 ounces each)
- 2 tablespoons extra virgin olive oil
- 1 lemon, thinly sliced
- 2 tablespoons fresh dill, chopped
- 2 cloves garlic, minced
- 1 teaspoon paprika
- 1/4 teaspoon ground black pepper
- Fresh dill sprigs for garnish (optional)

Instructions

1. Preheat Oven: Preheat your oven to 375°F (190°C). Line a baking sheet with parchment paper.
2. Prepare Salmon: Place the salmon fillets on the prepared baking sheet. Drizzle the olive oil over each fillet.
3. Add Lemon and Dill: Arrange the lemon slices on top of the salmon. Sprinkle with chopped dill, minced garlic, paprika, and black pepper.
4. Bake: Bake in the preheated oven for 18-20 minutes, or until the salmon flakes easily with a fork.
5. Serve: Garnish with fresh dill sprigs if desired and serve warm.

Nutrition Information (Per Serving)

- Calories: 330 kcal
- Protein: 35g
- Carbohydrates: 2g
- Fiber: 0g
- Sugars: 0g
- Fat: 20g
- Saturated Fat: 3g
- Sodium: 80mg

Cooking Time

- **Preparation Time: 10 minutes**
- **Cooking Time: 20 minutes**
- **Total Time: 30 minutes**

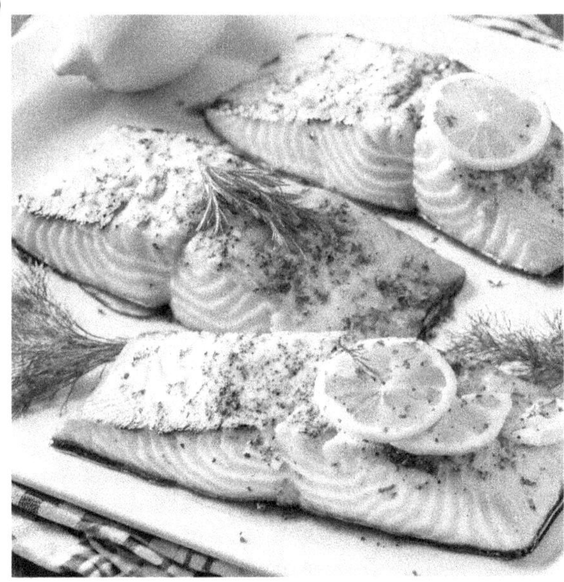

2. Grilled Tuna Steaks with Avocado Salsa

Ingredients (Serves 4)

- 4 tuna steaks (about 6 ounces each)
- 2 tablespoons olive oil
- 1 teaspoon ground cumin
- 1/2 teaspoon smoked paprika
- 1/4 teaspoon ground black pepper

Avocado Salsa:

- 1 ripe avocado, diced
- 1/2 cup cherry tomatoes, halved
- 1/4 cup red onion, finely chopped
- 1 tablespoon fresh lime juice
- 2 tablespoons fresh cilantro, chopped
- 1/4 teaspoon ground cumin

Instructions

1. Prepare Tuna: Brush the tuna steaks with olive oil and sprinkle with ground cumin, smoked paprika, and black pepper.
2. Preheat Grill: Preheat your grill or grill pan to medium-high heat.
3. Grill Tuna: Place the tuna steaks on the grill and cook for 3-4 minutes per side for medium-rare, or longer if desired. Remove from the grill and let rest for a few minutes.
4. Prepare Salsa: While the tuna is grilling, combine the diced avocado, cherry tomatoes, red onion, lime juice, cilantro, and cumin in a bowl. Gently mix until combined.
5. Serve: Top each grilled tuna steak with a generous spoonful of avocado salsa and serve immediately.

Nutrition Information (Per Serving)

- Calories: 370 kcal
- Protein: 40g
- Carbohydrates: 8g
- Fiber: 5g
- Sugars: 2g
- Fat: 20g
- Saturated Fat: 3g
- Sodium: 90mg

Cooking Time

- **Preparation Time: 10 minutes**
- **Cooking Time: 10 minutes**
- **Total Time: 20 minutes**

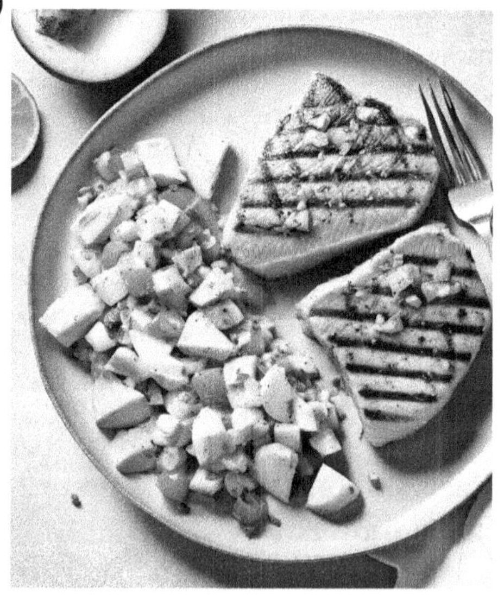

3. Shrimp and Quinoa Salad

Ingredients (Serves 4)

- 1 cup quinoa
- 2 cups water or low-sodium vegetable broth
- 1 pound large shrimp, peeled and deveined
- 2 tablespoons extra virgin olive oil
- 2 cloves garlic, minced
- 1 teaspoon paprika
- 1/2 teaspoon ground cumin
- 1 cup cherry tomatoes, halved
- 1 cucumber, diced
- 1/4 cup red onion, finely chopped
- 2 tablespoons fresh lemon juice
- 2 tablespoons fresh parsley, chopped

Instructions

1. Cook Quinoa: Rinse the quinoa under cold water. In a medium saucepan, combine quinoa and water (or vegetable broth). Bring to a boil, then reduce the heat to low, cover, and simmer for about 15 minutes, or until the quinoa is tender and the liquid is absorbed. Fluff with a fork and set aside to cool.
2. Cook Shrimp: In a large skillet, heat olive oil over medium heat. Add the minced garlic and cook for about 1 minute until fragrant. Add the shrimp, paprika, and cumin. Cook for 3-4 minutes until the shrimp are pink and opaque. Remove from heat.
3. Assemble Salad: In a large bowl, combine the cooked quinoa, shrimp, cherry tomatoes, cucumber, and red onion.
4. Dress Salad: Drizzle with fresh lemon juice and sprinkle with chopped parsley. Toss gently to combine.
5. Serve: Serve chilled or at room temperature.

Nutrition Information (Per Serving)

- Calories: 320 kcal Protein: 28g   Carbohydrates: 25g   Fiber: 5g
- Sugars: 3g
- Fat: 12g
- Saturated Fat: 2g
- Sodium: 250mg

Cooking Time

- **Preparation Time: 15 minutes**
- **Cooking Time: 20 minutes**
- **Total Time: 35 minutes**

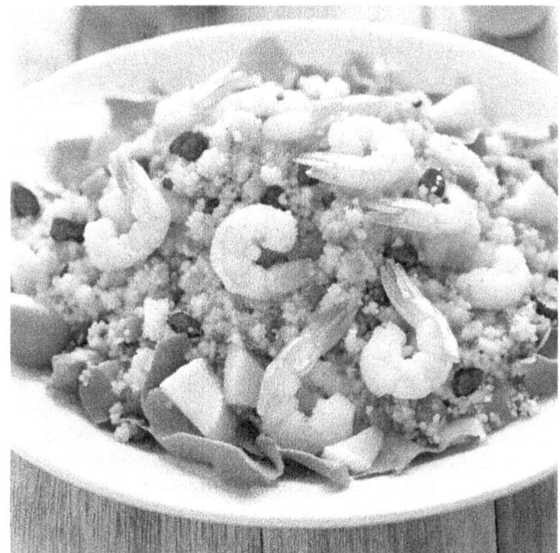

4. Garlic Butter Shrimp
Ingredients (Serves 4)

- 1 pound large shrimp, peeled and deveined
- 3 tablespoons unsalted butter
- 4 cloves garlic, minced
- 1 tablespoon fresh lemon juice
- 1/4 teaspoon ground black pepper
- 2 tablespoons fresh parsley, chopped
- Lemon wedges for serving (optional)

Instructions

1. Melt Butter: In a large skillet, melt the butter over medium heat.
2. Cook Garlic: Add the minced garlic and cook for 1-2 minutes until fragrant but not browned.
3. Cook Shrimp: Add the shrimp to the skillet and cook for about 2-3 minutes on each side until they are pink and opaque.
4. Add Lemon Juice and Seasoning: Stir in the fresh lemon juice and black pepper. Toss to coat the shrimp evenly.
5. Garnish and Serve: Remove from heat and sprinkle with chopped parsley. Serve warm with lemon wedges on the side, if desired.

Nutrition Information (Per Serving)

- Calories: 240 kcal
- Protein: 24g
- Carbohydrates: 3g
- Fiber: 0g
- Sugars: 0g
- Fat: 15g
- Saturated Fat: 8g
- Sodium: 180mg

Cooking Time

- **Preparation Time: 5 minutes**
- **Cooking Time: 10 minutes**
- **Total Time: 15 minutes**

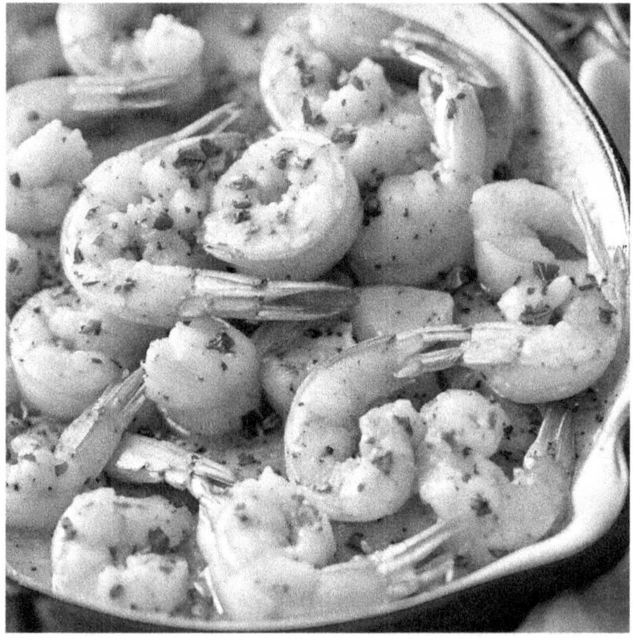

5. Miso Glazed Cod

Ingredients (Serves 4)

- 4 cod fillets (about 6 ounces each)
- 3 tablespoons white miso paste
- 2 tablespoons mirin (Japanese sweet rice wine)
- 1 tablespoon soy sauce (low-sodium)
- 1 tablespoon rice vinegar
- 1 tablespoon fresh ginger, grated
- 1 tablespoon honey or agave syrup
- 1 tablespoon sesame oil
- 2 green onions, finely sliced for garnish
- Sesame seeds for garnish (optional)

Instructions

1. Prepare Marinade: In a bowl, whisk together the miso paste, mirin, soy sauce, rice vinegar, grated ginger, honey, and sesame oil until smooth.
2. Marinate Cod: Place the cod fillets in a shallow dish and pour the marinade over them. Cover and refrigerate for at least 30 minutes, up to 2 hours.
3. Preheat Oven: Preheat your oven to 375°F (190°C). Line a baking sheet with parchment paper.
4. Bake Cod: Remove the cod from the marinade and place on the prepared baking sheet. Bake for 12-15 minutes, or until the fish is opaque and flakes easily with a fork.
5. Garnish and Serve: Garnish with sliced green onions and sesame seeds, if using. Serve immediately.

Nutrition Information (Per Serving)

- Calories: 260 kcal
- Protein: 33g
- Carbohydrates: 8g
- Fiber: 0g
- Sugars: 6g
- Fat: 9g
- Saturated Fat: 1g
- Sodium: 500mg

Cooking Time

- **Preparation Time: 10 minutes**
- **Marinating Time: 30 minutes**
- **Cooking Time: 15 minutes**

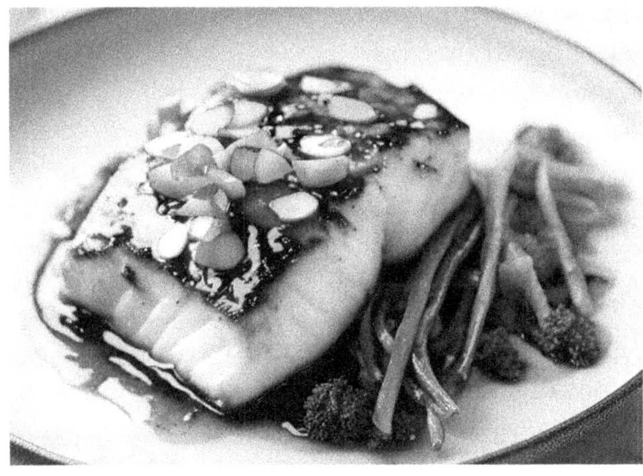

6. Seared Scallops with Spinach
Ingredients (Serves 4)

- 1 pound large sea scallops
- 2 tablespoons extra virgin olive oil
- 3 cloves garlic, minced
- 1/4 teaspoon ground black pepper
- 4 cups fresh spinach
- 1 tablespoon lemon juice
- 2 tablespoons fresh parsley, chopped

Instructions

1. Prepare Scallops: Pat the scallops dry with a paper towel. Season lightly with ground black pepper.
2. Heat Olive Oil: In a large skillet, heat 1 tablespoon of olive oil over medium-high heat.
3. Sear Scallops: Add the scallops to the skillet in a single layer, making sure they do not touch. Cook for 2-3 minutes on each side until golden brown and opaque. Remove from the skillet and set aside.
4. Sauté Garlic and Spinach: In the same skillet, add the remaining tablespoon of olive oil and minced garlic. Cook for 1 minute until fragrant, then add the spinach. Cook until wilted, about 2 minutes.
5. Finish with Lemon and Parsley: Return the scallops to the skillet and drizzle with lemon juice. Sprinkle with fresh parsley.
6. Serve: Serve immediately while warm.

Nutrition Information (Per Serving)

- Calories: 220 kcal
- Protein: 23g
- Carbohydrates: 5g
- Fiber: 2g
- Sugars: 1g
- Fat: 12g
- Saturated Fat: 2g
- Sodium: 400mg

Cooking Time

- **Preparation Time: 10 minutes**
- **Cooking Time: 10 minutes**
- **Total Time: 20 minutes**

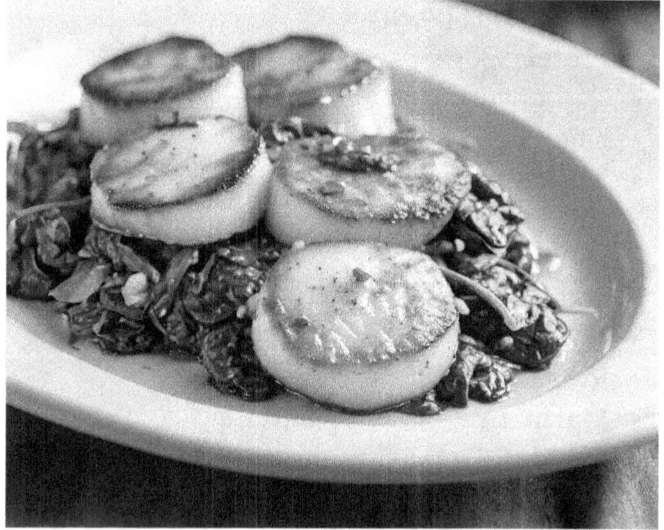

7. Mediterranean Baked Halibut

Ingredients (Serves 4)

- 4 halibut fillets (about 6 ounces each)
- 2 tablespoons extra virgin olive oil
- 2 tablespoons lemon juice
- 1 teaspoon dried oregano
- 1 teaspoon dried basil
- 1/4 teaspoon ground black pepper
- 1/2 cup cherry tomatoes, halved
- 1/4 cup Kalamata olives, pitted and halved
- 1/4 cup red onion, thinly sliced
- 2 tablespoons capers, drained
- Fresh basil leaves for garnish (optional)

Instructions

1. Preheat Oven: Preheat your oven to 400°F (200°C). Line a baking dish with parchment paper.
2. Prepare Marinade: In a small bowl, whisk together olive oil, lemon juice, dried oregano, dried basil, and black pepper.
3. Marinate Fish: Place the halibut fillets in the baking dish. Pour the marinade over the fish, ensuring they are well coated.
4. Add Vegetables: Scatter the cherry tomatoes, olives, red onion, and capers around the fish.
5. Bake: Bake in the preheated oven for 15-18 minutes, or until the fish is opaque and flakes easily with a fork.
6. Serve: Garnish with fresh basil leaves if desired and serve warm.

Nutrition Information (Per Serving)

- Calories: 300 kcal
- Protein: 35g
- Carbohydrates: 5g
- Fiber: 1g
- Sugars: 2g
- Fat: 16g
- Saturated Fat: 2g
- Sodium: 320mg

Cooking Time

- **Preparation Time: 10 minutes**
- **Cooking Time: 18 minutes**
- **Total Time: 28 minutes**

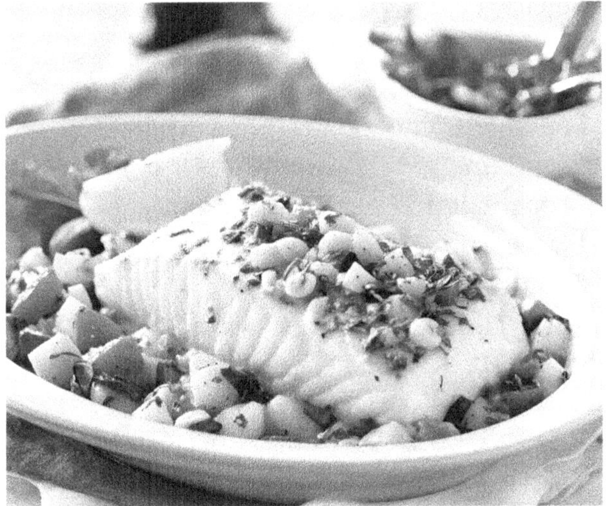

8. Lemon Herb Grilled Shrimp

Ingredients (Serves 4)

- 1 pound large shrimp, peeled and deveined
- 3 tablespoons extra virgin olive oil
- 2 tablespoons fresh lemon juice
- 2 teaspoons lemon zest
- 2 cloves garlic, minced
- 1 teaspoon dried oregano
- 1 teaspoon dried thyme
- 1/4 teaspoon ground black pepper
- Fresh parsley for garnish (optional)

Instructions

1. Prepare Marinade: In a bowl, whisk together the olive oil, lemon juice, lemon zest, garlic, dried oregano, dried thyme, and black pepper.
2. Marinate Shrimp: Add the shrimp to the bowl and toss to coat. Cover and refrigerate for 15-30 minutes.
3. Preheat Grill: Preheat your grill or grill pan to medium-high heat.
4. Grill Shrimp: Thread the shrimp onto skewers (if using) and grill for 2-3 minutes on each side, until they are pink and opaque.
5. Serve: Remove from the grill and garnish with fresh parsley if desired. Serve warm.

Nutrition Information (Per Serving)

- Calories: 220 kcal
- Protein: 24g
- Carbohydrates: 2g
- Fiber: 0g
- Sugars: 0g
- Fat: 12g
- Saturated Fat: 2g
- Sodium: 180mg

Cooking Time

- **Preparation Time: 10 minutes**
- **Marinating Time: 15 minutes**
- **Cooking Time: 6 minutes**
- **Total Time: 31 minutes**

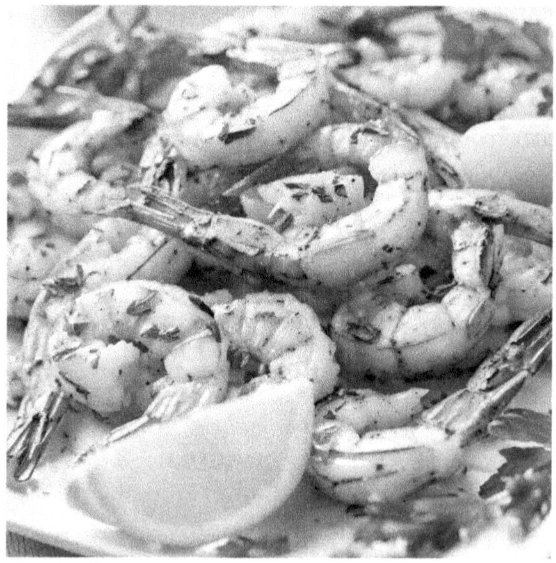

9. Salmon and Asparagus Foil Packets

Ingredients (Serves 4)

- 4 salmon fillets (about 6 ounces each)
- 1 pound asparagus, trimmed
- 4 tablespoons extra virgin olive oil
- 2 tablespoons fresh lemon juice
- 1 tablespoon lemon zest
- 2 cloves garlic, minced
- 1 teaspoon dried dill
- 1/4 teaspoon ground black pepper
- Fresh parsley or dill for garnish (optional)

Instructions

1. Preheat Oven: Preheat your oven to 375°F (190°C). Cut four pieces of aluminum foil, each large enough to wrap a salmon fillet and asparagus.
2. Prepare Marinade: In a small bowl, whisk together the olive oil, lemon juice, lemon zest, garlic, dried dill, and black pepper.
3. Assemble Packets: Place a salmon fillet in the center of each piece of foil. Arrange asparagus spears around the salmon. Drizzle the marinade evenly over the salmon and asparagus.
4. Seal Packets: Fold the sides of the foil up and over the salmon and asparagus to create a sealed packet.
5. Bake: Place the foil packets on a baking sheet and bake in the preheated oven for 20-25 minutes, or until the salmon is opaque and flakes easily with a fork.
6. Serve: Open the packets carefully and garnish with fresh parsley or dill if desired. Serve warm.

Nutrition Information (Per Serving)

- Calories: 330 kcal
- Protein: 35g
- Carbohydrates: 5g
- Fiber: 2g
- Sugars: 2g
- Fat: 18g
- Saturated Fat: 3g
- Sodium: 90mg

Cooking Time

- **Preparation Time: 10 minutes**
- **Cooking Time: 25 minutes**
- **Total Time: 35 minutes**

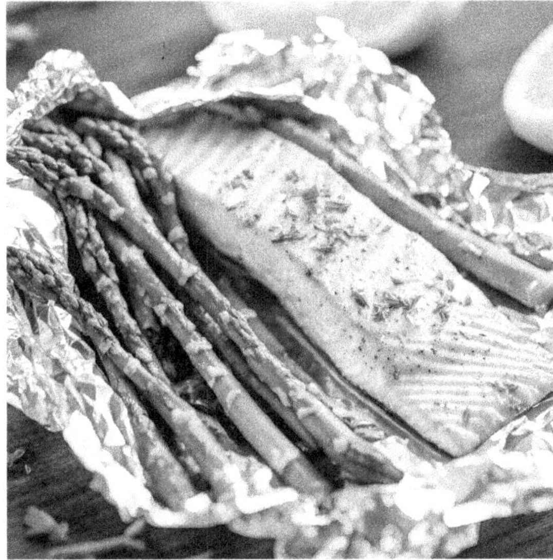

10. Tuna Salad with White Beans and Arugula

Ingredients (Serves 4)

- 2 cans (5 ounces each) tuna packed in water, drained
- 1 can (15 ounces) white beans (cannellini or great northern), rinsed and drained
- 4 cups arugula
- 1/2 cup cherry tomatoes, halved
- 1/4 cup red onion, thinly sliced
- 2 tablespoons capers, drained
- 3 tablespoons extra virgin olive oil
- 2 tablespoons fresh lemon juice
- 1 teaspoon Dijon mustard
- 1/4 teaspoon ground black pepper

Instructions

1. Prepare Salad Base: In a large bowl, combine the tuna, white beans, arugula, cherry tomatoes, red onion, and capers.
2. Make Dressing: In a small bowl, whisk together the olive oil, lemon juice, Dijon mustard, and black pepper.
3. Toss Salad: Pour the dressing over the salad and toss gently to combine.
4. Serve: Divide the salad into four servings and serve immediately.

Nutrition Information (Per Serving)

- Calories: 280 kcal
- Protein: 24g
- Carbohydrates: 18g
- Fiber: 5g
- Sugars: 2g
- Fat: 14g
- Saturated Fat: 2g
- Sodium: 400mg

Cooking Time

- **Preparation Time: 10 minutes**
- **Total Time: 10 minutes**

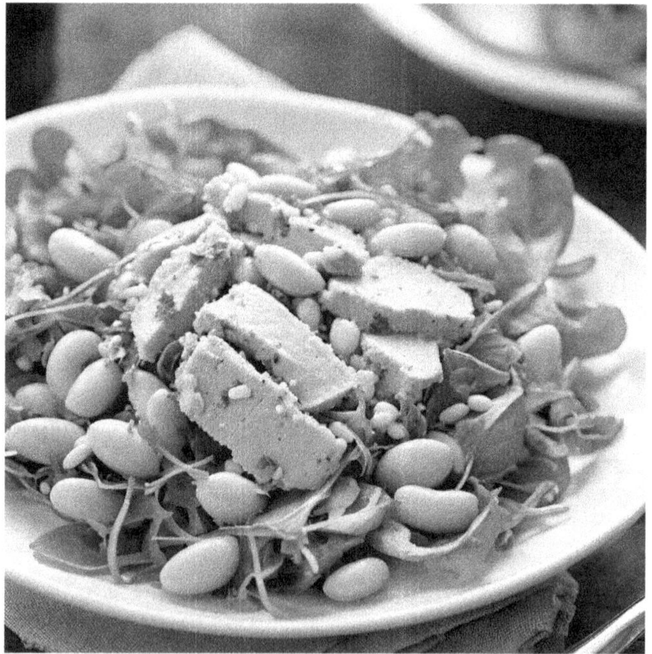

11. Spicy Baked Cod

Ingredients (Serves 4)

- 4 cod fillets (about 6 ounces each)
- 2 tablespoons extra virgin olive oil
- 2 tablespoons lemon juice
- 1 tablespoon paprika
- 1 teaspoon ground cumin
- 1/2 teaspoon ground coriander
- 1/4 teaspoon ground black pepper
- 1/4 teaspoon red pepper flakes
- 2 cloves garlic, minced
- Fresh cilantro for garnish (optional)
- Lemon wedges for serving (optional)

Instructions

1. Preheat Oven: Preheat your oven to 375°F (190°C). Line a baking sheet with parchment paper.
2. Prepare Marinade: In a small bowl, whisk together olive oil, lemon juice, paprika, cumin, coriander, black pepper, red pepper flakes, and minced garlic.
3. Marinate Cod: Place the cod fillets on the prepared baking sheet. Brush or spoon the marinade evenly over each fillet.
4. Bake Cod: Bake in the preheated oven for 15-20 minutes, or until the fish is opaque and flakes easily with a fork.
5. Serve: Garnish with fresh cilantro and serve with lemon wedges if desired. Serve warm.

Nutrition Information (Per Serving)

- Calories: 220 kcal
- Protein: 33g
- Carbohydrates: 2g
- Fiber: 1g
- Sugars: 0g
- Fat: 9g
- Saturated Fat: 1g
- Sodium: 80mg

Cooking Time

- **Preparation Time: 10 minutes**
- **Cooking Time: 20 minutes**
- **Total Time: 30 minutes**

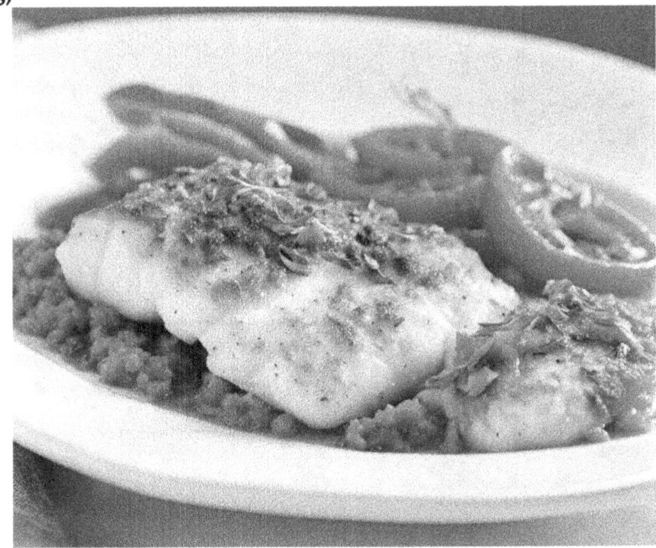

12. Garlic Lemon Shrimp Pasta

Ingredients (Serves 4)

- 8 ounces whole grain or gluten-free pasta
- 1 pound large shrimp, peeled and deveined
- 3 tablespoons extra virgin olive oil
- 4 cloves garlic, minced
- 1/4 teaspoon red pepper flakes
- 1/4 teaspoon ground black pepper
- 1 lemon, zested and juiced
- 1/4 cup fresh parsley, chopped
- 1/4 cup grated Parmesan cheese (optional)

Instructions

1. Cook Pasta: Bring a large pot of water to a boil and cook the pasta according to package instructions until al dente. Drain and set aside.
2. Cook Shrimp: In a large skillet, heat the olive oil over medium heat. Add the minced garlic and red pepper flakes, and cook for about 1 minute until fragrant.
3. Add Shrimp: Add the shrimp to the skillet and cook for 2-3 minutes on each side until they are pink and opaque. Remove the shrimp from the skillet and set aside.
4. Combine Ingredients: Add the cooked pasta to the skillet. Stir in the lemon zest, lemon juice, and black pepper. Toss to combine.
5. Add Shrimp and Garnish: Return the shrimp to the skillet and toss gently to combine. Sprinkle with fresh parsley and Parmesan cheese, if using.
6. Serve: Serve warm.

Nutrition Information (Per Serving)

- Calories: 360 kcal
- Protein: 27g
- Carbohydrates: 45g
- Fiber: 6g
- Sugars: 3g
- Fat: 10g
- Saturated Fat: 2g
- Sodium: 300mg

Cooking Time

- **Preparation Time: 10 minutes**
- **Cooking Time: 15 minutes**
- **Total Time: 25 minutes**

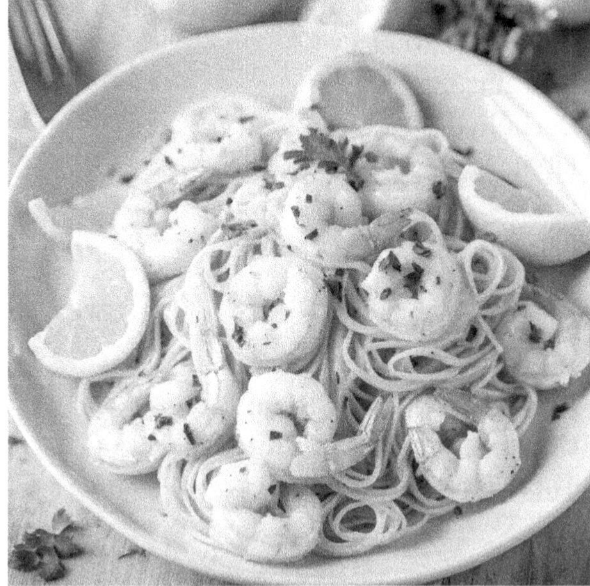

13. Citrus Marinated Salmon

Ingredients (Serves 4)

- 4 salmon fillets (about 6 ounces each)
- 1/4 cup orange juice
- 2 tablespoons lemon juice
- 2 tablespoons lime juice
- 2 tablespoons olive oil
- 1 tablespoon honey or agave syrup
- 1 tablespoon fresh ginger, grated
- 1/2 teaspoon ground coriander
- 1/4 teaspoon ground black pepper
- Fresh cilantro or mint for garnish (optional)

Instructions

1. Prepare Marinade: In a small bowl, whisk together orange juice, lemon juice, lime juice, olive oil, honey, grated ginger, ground coriander, and black pepper.
2. Marinate Salmon: Place the salmon fillets in a shallow dish and pour the marinade over them. Cover and refrigerate for at least 30 minutes, up to 2 hours.
3. Preheat Oven: Preheat your oven to 375°F (190°C). Line a baking sheet with parchment paper.
4. Bake Salmon: Remove the salmon from the marinade and place on the prepared baking sheet. Bake for 15-20 minutes, or until the salmon is opaque and flakes easily with a fork.
5. Serve: Garnish with fresh cilantro or mint if desired. Serve warm.

Nutrition Information (Per Serving)

- Calories: 320 kcal
- Protein: 35g
- Carbohydrates: 8g
- Fiber: 1g
- Sugars: 6g
- Fat: 16g
- Saturated Fat: 3g
- Sodium: 100mg

Cooking Time

- **Preparation Time: 10 minutes**
- **Marinating Time: 30 minutes**
- **Cooking Time: 20 minutes**
- **Total Time: 60 minutes**

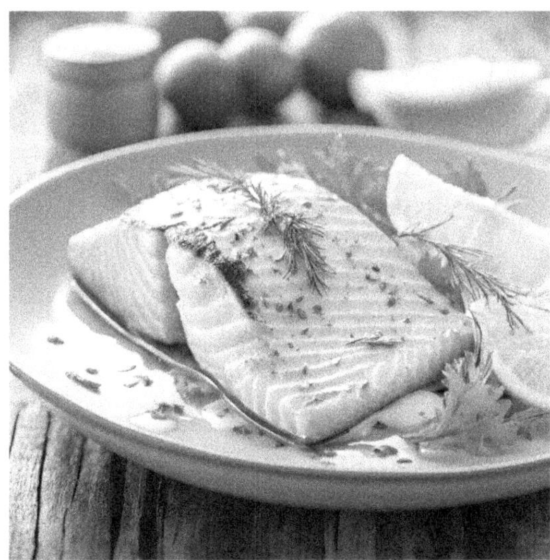

14. Grilled Mahi Mahi with Mango Salsa
Ingredients (Serves 4)

- 4 mahi mahi fillets (about 6 ounces each)
- 2 tablespoons extra virgin olive oil
- 2 tablespoons lime juice
- 1 teaspoon ground cumin
- 1/4 teaspoon ground black pepper

Mango Salsa:

- 1 ripe mango, peeled and diced
- 1/2 red bell pepper, diced
- 1/4 cup red onion, finely chopped
- 1 jalapeño, seeded and finely chopped
- 2 tablespoons fresh cilantro, chopped
- 1 tablespoon lime juice

Instructions

1. Prepare Marinade: In a small bowl, whisk together olive oil, lime juice, ground cumin, and black pepper.
2. Marinate Fish: Brush the mahi mahi fillets with the marinade and let sit for 10 minutes.
3. Prepare Salsa: In a medium bowl, combine the diced mango, red bell pepper, red onion, jalapeño, cilantro, and lime juice. Mix well and set aside.
4. Preheat Grill: Preheat your grill or grill pan to medium-high heat.
5. Grill Mahi Mahi: Grill the mahi mahi fillets for about 4-5 minutes on each side, or until they are opaque and flake easily with a fork.
6. Serve: Top the grilled mahi mahi with the mango salsa and serve warm.

Nutrition Information (Per Serving)

- Calories: 290 kcal
- Protein: 30g
- Carbohydrates: 15g
- Fiber: 3g
- Sugars: 10g (natural sugars from mango)
- Fat: 12g
- Saturated Fat: 2g
- Sodium: 140mg

Cooking Time

- **Preparation Time: 15 minutes**
- **Cooking Time: 10 minutes**
- **Total Time: 25 minutes**

15. Salmon and Sweet Potato Cakes

Ingredients (Serves 4)

- 1 pound cooked salmon, flaked
- 1 cup cooked sweet potato, mashed
- 1/4 cup green onion, finely chopped
- 1/4 cup fresh parsley, chopped
- 1 egg, beaten
- 2 tablespoons almond flour
- 1 tablespoon Dijon mustard
- 1 teaspoon smoked paprika
- 1/4 teaspoon ground black pepper
- 2 tablespoons extra virgin olive oil
- Lemon wedges for serving (optional)

Instructions

1. Prepare Mixture: In a large bowl, combine the flaked salmon, mashed sweet potato, green onion, parsley, beaten egg, almond flour, Dijon mustard, smoked paprika, and black pepper. Mix until well combined.
2. Form Patties: Shape the mixture into 8 patties.
3. Heat Oil: Heat the olive oil in a large skillet over medium heat.
4. Cook Patties: Cook the patties in the skillet for about 3-4 minutes on each side, or until golden brown and heated through.
5. Serve: Serve the salmon cakes warm with lemon wedges if desired.

Nutrition Information (Per Serving)

- Calories: 310 kcal
- Protein: 28g
- Carbohydrates: 15g
- Fiber: 3g
- Sugars: 4g (natural sugars from sweet potato)
- Fat: 16g
- Saturated Fat: 3g
- Sodium: 240mg

Cooking Time

- **Preparation Time: 15 minutes**
- **Cooking Time: 10 minutes**
- **Total Time: 25 minutes**

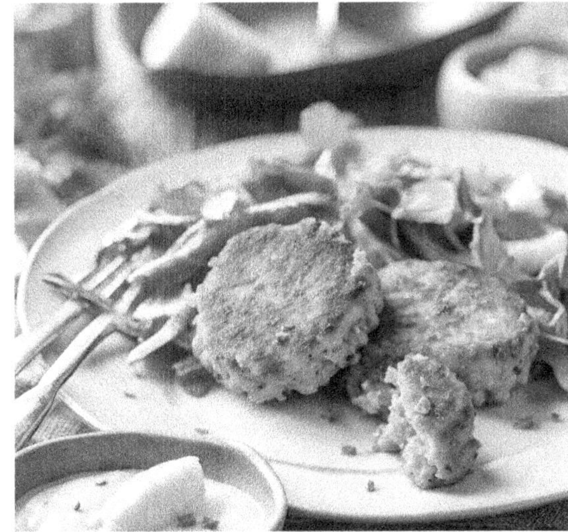

16. Steamed Mussels with Garlic and Parsley

Ingredients (Serves 4)

- 2 pounds fresh mussels, cleaned and debearded
- 2 tablespoons extra virgin olive oil
- 4 cloves garlic, minced
- 1 cup dry white wine or vegetable broth
- 2 tablespoons fresh lemon juice
- 1/4 teaspoon ground black pepper
- 1/4 cup fresh parsley, chopped
- Lemon wedges for serving (optional)

Instructions

1. Prepare Mussels: Ensure the mussels are cleaned and debearded. Discard any that are open and do not close when tapped.
2. Heat Oil: In a large pot or Dutch oven, heat the olive oil over medium heat.
3. Cook Garlic: Add the minced garlic and cook for about 1 minute until fragrant.
4. Add Liquid: Pour in the white wine (or vegetable broth) and lemon juice. Bring to a simmer.
5. Steam Mussels: Add the mussels to the pot and cover with a lid. Cook for about 5-7 minutes, shaking the pot occasionally, until the mussels open. Discard any that do not open.
6. Finish with Seasoning: Sprinkle with ground black pepper and chopped parsley.
7. Serve: Serve the steamed mussels with lemon wedges if desired.

Nutrition Information (Per Serving)

- Calories: 220 kcal
- Protein: 30g
- Carbohydrates: 4g
- Fiber: 1g
- Sugars: 1g
- Fat: 8g
- Saturated Fat: 1g
- Sodium: 400mg

Cooking Time

- **Preparation Time: 10 minutes**
- **Cooking Time: 10 minutes**
- **Total Time: 20 minutes**

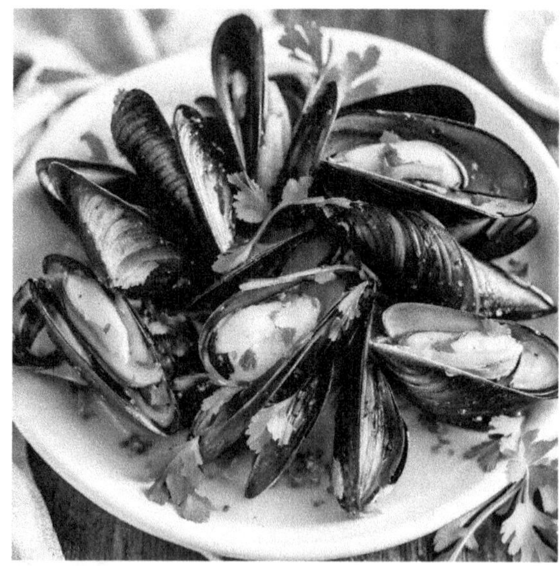

17. Tuna and Avocado Salad

Ingredients (Serves 4)

- 2 cans (5 ounces each) tuna packed in water, drained
- 2 ripe avocados, diced
- 1 cup cherry tomatoes, halved
- 1/4 cup red onion, finely chopped
- 1/4 cup fresh cilantro, chopped
- 2 tablespoons fresh lime juice
- 2 tablespoons extra virgin olive oil
- 1/4 teaspoon ground black pepper

Instructions

1. Prepare Ingredients: In a large bowl, combine the drained tuna, diced avocados, cherry tomatoes, red onion, and cilantro.
2. Mix Dressing: In a small bowl, whisk together the lime juice, olive oil, and black pepper.
3. Combine: Pour the dressing over the tuna mixture and toss gently to combine.
4. Serve: Divide the salad into four servings. Serve immediately.

Nutrition Information (Per Serving)

- Calories: 320 kcal
- Protein: 22g
- Carbohydrates: 12g
- Fiber: 8g
- Sugars: 2g
- Fat: 22g
- Saturated Fat: 3g
- Sodium: 250mg

Cooking Time

- **Preparation Time: 10 minutes**
- **Total Time: 10 minutes**

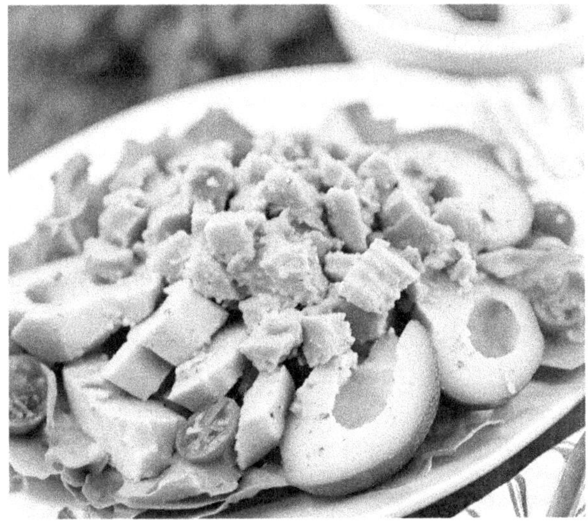

18. Baked Sole with Lemon and Capers

Ingredients (Serves 4)

- 4 sole fillets (about 6 ounces each)
- 2 tablespoons extra virgin olive oil
- 1 lemon, thinly sliced
- 2 tablespoons fresh lemon juice
- 2 tablespoons capers, rinsed and drained
- 1 teaspoon fresh dill, chopped
- 1/4 teaspoon ground black pepper

Instructions

1. Preheat Oven: Preheat your oven to 375°F (190°C). Line a baking sheet with parchment paper.
2. Prepare Fish: Place the sole fillets on the prepared baking sheet. Drizzle with olive oil and lemon juice. Sprinkle with ground black pepper.
3. Add Lemon and Capers: Arrange the lemon slices on top of the fillets and scatter the capers around them.
4. Bake: Bake in the preheated oven for 12-15 minutes, or until the fish is opaque and flakes easily with a fork.
5. Garnish and Serve: Sprinkle with fresh dill and serve immediately.

Nutrition Information (Per Serving)

- Calories: 200 kcal
- Protein: 28g
- Carbohydrates: 2g
- Fiber: 1g
- Sugars: 0g
- Fat: 8g
- Saturated Fat: 1g
- Sodium: 220mg

Cooking Time

- **Preparation Time: 10 minutes**
- **Cooking Time: 15 minutes**
- **Total Time: 25 minutes**

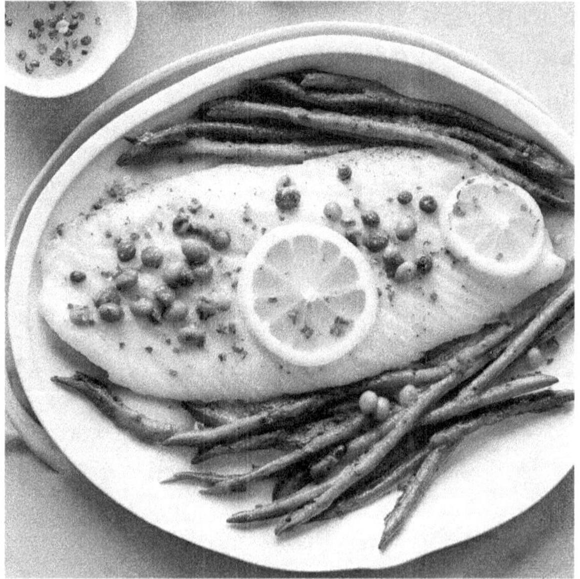

19. Lemon Dill Baked Haddock

Ingredients (Serves 4)

- 4 haddock fillets (about 6 ounces each)
- 2 tablespoons extra virgin olive oil
- 2 tablespoons fresh lemon juice
- 1 tablespoon lemon zest
- 1 tablespoon fresh dill, chopped
- 1/4 teaspoon ground black pepper
- Lemon wedges for serving (optional)

Instructions

1. Preheat Oven: Preheat your oven to 375°F (190°C). Line a baking dish with parchment paper.
2. Prepare Marinade: In a small bowl, mix together the olive oil, lemon juice, lemon zest, chopped dill, and black pepper.
3. Marinate Fish: Place the haddock fillets in the baking dish. Pour the marinade over the fillets, making sure they are well coated.
4. Bake: Bake in the preheated oven for 15-18 minutes, or until the fish is opaque and flakes easily with a fork.
5. Serve: Serve warm with lemon wedges if desired.

Nutrition Information (Per Serving)

- Calories: 230 kcal
- Protein: 34g
- Carbohydrates: 2g
- Fiber: 0g
- Sugars: 0g
- Fat: 10g
- Saturated Fat: 2g
- Sodium: 110mg

Cooking Time

- **Preparation Time: 10 minutes**
- **Cooking Time: 18 minutes**
- **Total Time: 28 minutes**

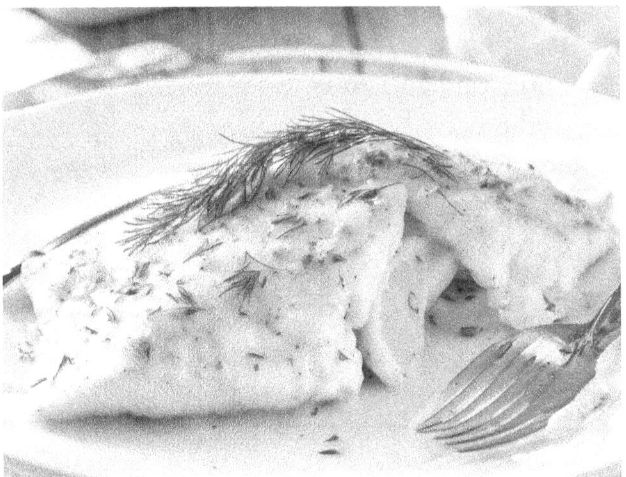

20. Tuna and Olive Tapenade Wraps
Ingredients (Serves 4)
- 2 cans (5 ounces each) tuna packed in water, drained
- 1/2 cup black olive tapenade
- 4 whole grain tortillas
- 1 cup arugula
- 1/2 cup cherry tomatoes, halved
- 1/4 cup red onion, thinly sliced
- 1 tablespoon fresh lemon juice
- 2 tablespoons extra virgin olive oil

Instructions
1. Prepare Filling: In a bowl, combine the drained tuna and black olive tapenade.
2. Assemble Wraps: Lay out the tortillas and divide the tuna mixture evenly among them. Top with arugula, cherry tomatoes, and red onion.
3. Add Dressing: Drizzle each wrap with lemon juice and olive oil.
4. Wrap: Roll up the tortillas tightly and slice in half if desired.
5. Serve: Serve immediately.

Nutrition Information (Per Serving)
- Calories: 340 kcal
- Protein: 23g
- Carbohydrates: 30g
- Fiber: 5g
- Sugars: 2g
- Fat: 15g
- Saturated Fat: 2g
- Sodium: 540mg

Cooking Time
- **Preparation Time: 10 minutes**
- **Total Time: 10 minutes**

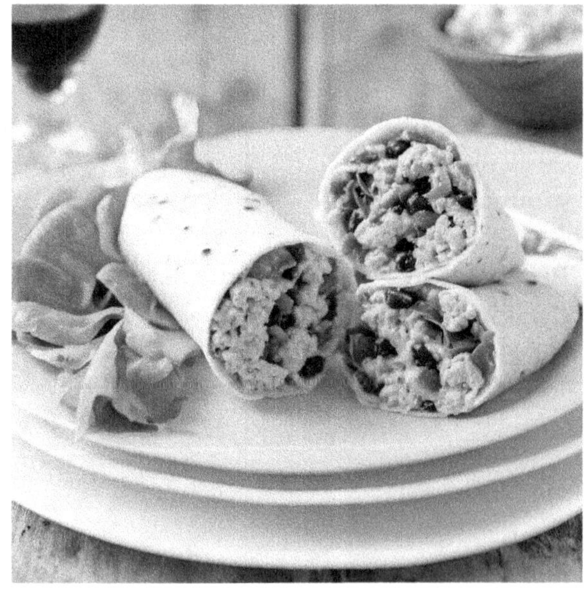

21. Ginger Soy Glazed Salmon

Ingredients (Serves 4)

- 4 salmon fillets (about 6 ounces each)
- 1/4 cup low-sodium soy sauce
- 2 tablespoons honey or agave syrup
- 1 tablespoon fresh ginger, grated
- 1 tablespoon rice vinegar
- 1 tablespoon sesame oil
- 2 cloves garlic, minced
- 1/4 teaspoon ground black pepper
- 1 tablespoon sesame seeds for garnish (optional)
- 2 green onions, thinly sliced for garnish (optional)

Instructions

1. Prepare Marinade: In a bowl, whisk together the soy sauce, honey, grated ginger, rice vinegar, sesame oil, minced garlic, and black pepper.
2. Marinate Salmon: Place the salmon fillets in a shallow dish and pour the marinade over them. Cover and refrigerate for at least 30 minutes, up to 2 hours.
3. Preheat Oven: Preheat your oven to 375°F (190°C). Line a baking sheet with parchment paper.
4. Bake Salmon: Remove the salmon from the marinade and place on the prepared baking sheet. Bake for 15-20 minutes, or until the salmon is opaque and flakes easily with a fork.
5. Garnish and Serve: Sprinkle with sesame seeds and sliced green onions if desired. Serve warm.

Nutrition Information (Per Serving)

- Calories: 340 kcal
- Protein: 34g
- Carbohydrates: 10g
- Fiber: 0g
- Sugars: 7g
- Fat: 18g
- Saturated Fat: 3g
- Sodium: 420mg

Cooking Time

- **Preparation Time: 10 minutes**
- **Marinating Time: 30 minutes**
- **Cooking Time: 20 minutes**
- **Total Time: 60 minutes**

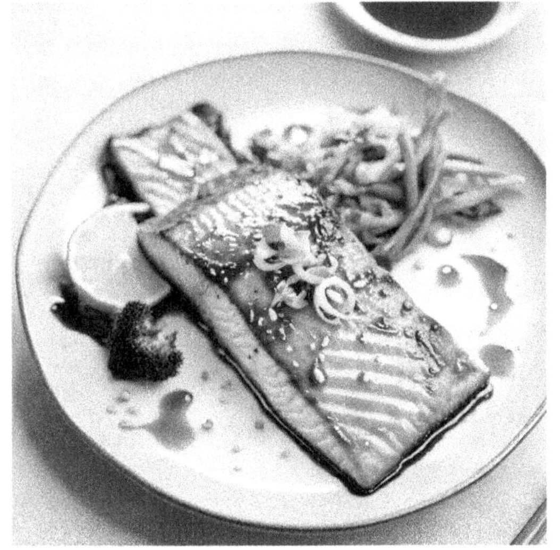

22. Broiled Lemon Garlic Fish
Ingredients (Serves 4)

- 4 white fish fillets (such as tilapia, haddock, or cod, about 6 ounces each)
- 3 tablespoons extra virgin olive oil
- 2 cloves garlic, minced
- 2 tablespoons fresh lemon juice
- 1 tablespoon lemon zest
- 1/4 teaspoon ground black pepper
- Fresh parsley for garnish (optional)
- Lemon wedges for serving (optional)

Instructions

1. Preheat Broiler: Preheat your oven's broiler to high. Line a broiler pan with aluminum foil.
2. Prepare Marinade: In a small bowl, mix together the olive oil, minced garlic, lemon juice, lemon zest, and black pepper.
3. Marinate Fish: Place the fish fillets on the broiler pan. Brush or spoon the marinade over each fillet.
4. Broil Fish: Broil the fish for 4-6 minutes on each side, or until the fish is opaque and flakes easily with a fork. The exact time will depend on the thickness of the fillets.
5. Serve: Garnish with fresh parsley and serve with lemon wedges if desired. Serve warm.

Nutrition Information (Per Serving)

- Calories: 260 kcal
- Protein: 34g
- Carbohydrates: 2g
- Fiber: 0g
- Sugars: 0g
- Fat: 12g
- Saturated Fat: 2g
- Sodium: 150mg

Cooking Time

- **Preparation Time: 10 minutes**
- **Cooking Time: 12 minutes**
- **Total Time: 22 minutes**

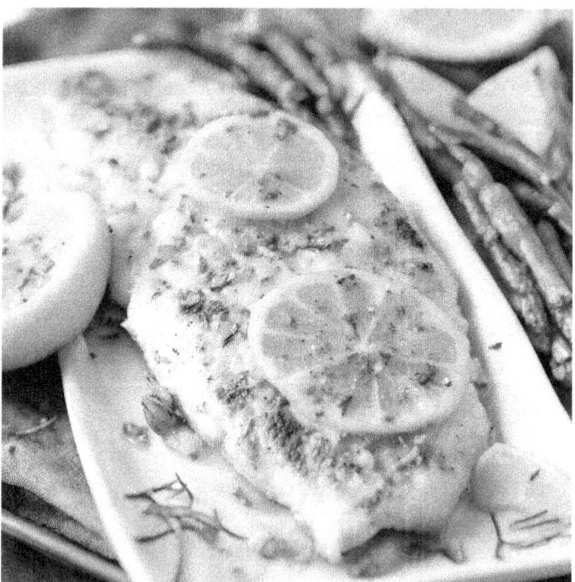

23. Shrimp and Zucchini Noodles

Ingredients (Serves 4)

- 1 pound large shrimp, peeled and deveined
- 4 medium zucchini, spiralized into noodles
- 3 tablespoons extra virgin olive oil
- 3 cloves garlic, minced
- 1/4 teaspoon red pepper flakes
- 1 tablespoon fresh lemon juice
- 1/4 teaspoon ground black pepper
- 1/4 cup fresh parsley, chopped
- Lemon wedges for serving (optional)

Instructions

1. Cook Shrimp: In a large skillet, heat 1 tablespoon of olive oil over medium heat. Add the shrimp, minced garlic, red pepper flakes, and black pepper. Cook for 2-3 minutes on each side until the shrimp are pink and opaque. Remove from the skillet and set aside.
2. Cook Zucchini Noodles: In the same skillet, heat the remaining 2 tablespoons of olive oil. Add the spiralized zucchini noodles and cook for 2-3 minutes, tossing frequently until just tender.
3. Combine and Heat: Return the shrimp to the skillet. Add the lemon juice and toss everything together. Cook for an additional 1-2 minutes to heat through.
4. Serve: Divide into four servings, garnish with fresh parsley, and serve with lemon wedges if desired.

Nutrition Information (Per Serving)

- Calories: 220 kcal
- Protein: 23g
- Carbohydrates: 8g
- Fiber: 2g
- Sugars: 5g (natural sugars from zucchini)
- Fat: 12g
- Saturated Fat: 2g
- Sodium: 250mg

Cooking Time

- **Preparation Time: 10 minutes**
- **Cooking Time: 10 minutes**
- **Total Time: 20 minutes**

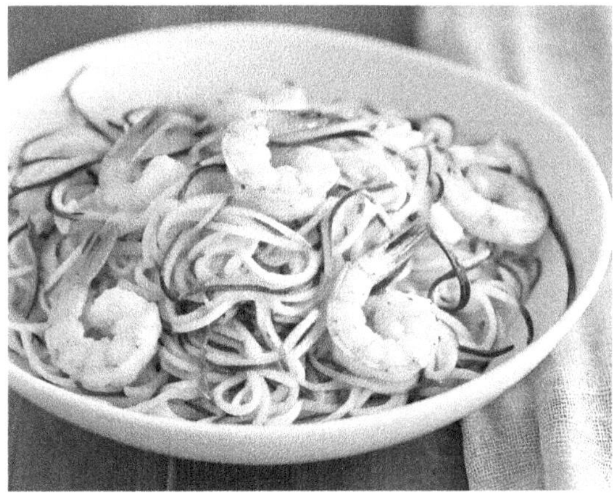

24. Baked Trout with Almonds
Ingredients (Serves 4)
- 4 trout fillets (about 6 ounces each)
- 2 tablespoons extra virgin olive oil
- 1/4 cup sliced almonds
- 2 tablespoons fresh lemon juice
- 1 tablespoon fresh parsley, chopped
- 1/4 teaspoon ground black pepper
- Lemon wedges for serving (optional)

Instructions
1. Preheat Oven: Preheat your oven to 375°F (190°C). Line a baking sheet with parchment paper.
2. Prepare Fish: Place the trout fillets on the prepared baking sheet. Drizzle with olive oil and lemon juice. Sprinkle with black pepper.
3. Add Almonds: Sprinkle the sliced almonds evenly over the trout fillets.
4. Bake: Bake in the preheated oven for 15-18 minutes, or until the trout is opaque and flakes easily with a fork.
5. Serve: Garnish with fresh parsley and serve with lemon wedges if desired. Serve warm.

Nutrition Information (Per Serving)
- Calories: 290 kcal
- Protein: 35g
- Carbohydrates: 3g
- Fiber: 1g
- Sugars: 0g
- Fat: 16g
- Saturated Fat: 3g
- Sodium: 110mg

Cooking Time
- **Preparation Time: 10 minutes**
- **Cooking Time: 18 minutes**
- **Total Time: 28 minutes**

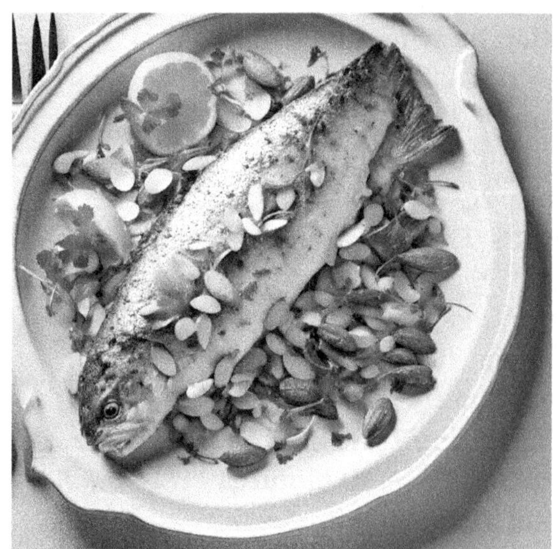

25. Clam and Kale Soup

Ingredients (Serves 4)

- 1 pound fresh clams, cleaned
- 2 tablespoons extra virgin olive oil
- 1 medium onion, finely chopped
- 3 cloves garlic, minced
- 4 cups low-sodium vegetable broth
- 1 cup diced tomatoes (canned, no salt added)
- 2 cups chopped kale, stems removed
- 1/4 teaspoon ground black pepper
- 1/4 teaspoon red pepper flakes
- 1 tablespoon fresh parsley, chopped

Instructions

1. Cook Aromatics: In a large pot, heat the olive oil over medium heat. Add the onion and garlic and cook until softened, about 5 minutes.
2. Add Broth and Tomatoes: Stir in the vegetable broth and diced tomatoes. Bring to a simmer.
3. Cook Clams: Add the clams to the pot. Cover and cook for about 5-7 minutes, or until the clams open. Discard any that do not open.
4. Add Kale and Seasoning: Stir in the chopped kale, black pepper, and red pepper flakes. Cook for another 2-3 minutes until the kale is wilted.
5. Serve: Ladle the soup into bowls, garnish with fresh parsley, and serve warm.

Nutrition Information (Per Serving)

- Calories: 200 kcal
- Protein: 16g
- Carbohydrates: 16g
- Fiber: 4g
- Sugars: 4g (natural sugars from tomatoes)
- Fat: 8g
- Saturated Fat: 1g
- Sodium: 400mg

Cooking Time

- **Preparation Time: 10 minutes**
- **Cooking Time: 20 minutes**
- **Total Time: 30 minutes**

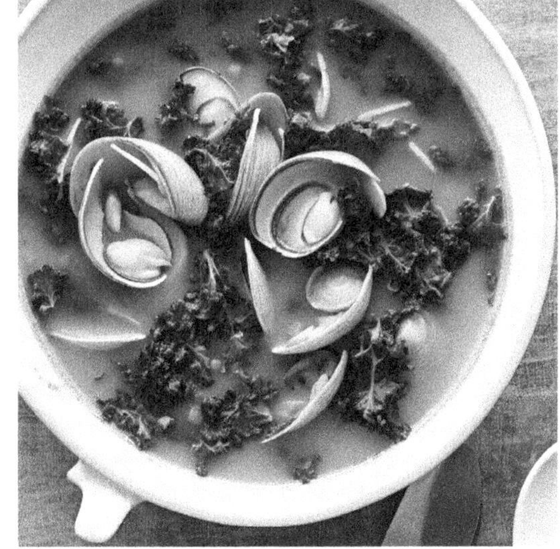

26. Baked Tilapia with Tomatoes and Basil

Ingredients (Serves 4)

- 4 tilapia fillets (about 6 ounces each)
- 2 tablespoons extra virgin olive oil
- 1 cup cherry tomatoes, halved
- 1/4 cup fresh basil, chopped
- 2 tablespoons fresh lemon juice
- 1/4 teaspoon ground black pepper
- Lemon wedges for serving (optional)

Instructions

1. Preheat Oven: Preheat your oven to 375°F (190°C). Line a baking dish with parchment paper.
2. Prepare Fish: Place the tilapia fillets in the baking dish. Drizzle with olive oil and lemon juice. Sprinkle with black pepper.
3. Add Toppings: Scatter the cherry tomatoes and chopped basil over the fillets.
4. Bake: Bake in the preheated oven for 15-18 minutes, or until the fish is opaque and flakes easily with a fork.
5. Serve: Serve warm with lemon wedges if desired.

Nutrition Information (Per Serving)

- Calories: 220 kcal
- Protein: 30g
- Carbohydrates: 4g
- Fiber: 1g
- Sugars: 2g (natural sugars from tomatoes)
- Fat: 10g
- Saturated Fat: 2g
- Sodium: 100mg

Cooking Time

- **Preparation Time: 10 minutes**
- **Cooking Time: 18 minutes**
- **Total Time: 28 minutes**

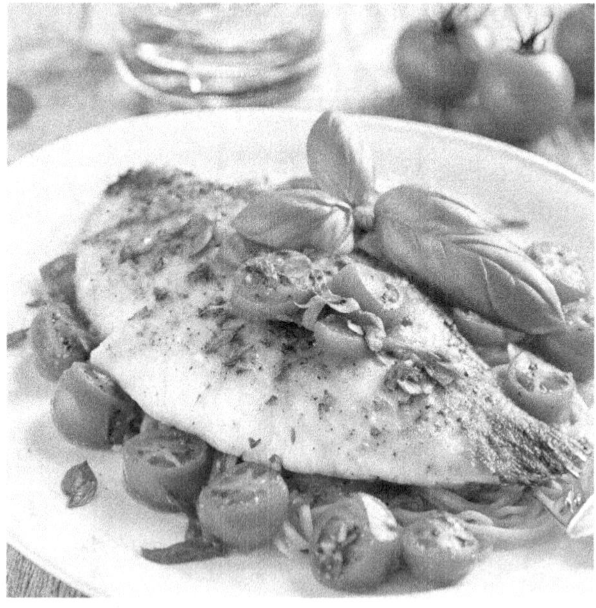

27. Shrimp and Avocado Rice Bowls

Ingredients (Serves 4)

- 1 pound large shrimp, peeled and deveined
- 2 tablespoons extra virgin olive oil
- 1 tablespoon fresh lime juice
- 1 teaspoon ground cumin
- 1/4 teaspoon ground black pepper
- 2 cups cooked brown rice
- 1 ripe avocado, diced
- 1 cup cherry tomatoes, halved
- 1/4 cup red onion, finely chopped
- 1/4 cup fresh cilantro, chopped

Instructions

1. Cook Shrimp: In a skillet, heat the olive oil over medium heat. Add the shrimp, lime juice, ground cumin, and black pepper. Cook for 2-3 minutes on each side until the shrimp are pink and opaque. Remove from heat.
2. Assemble Bowls: Divide the cooked brown rice into four bowls. Top with cooked shrimp, diced avocado, cherry tomatoes, and red onion.
3. Garnish: Sprinkle with fresh cilantro.
4. Serve: Serve immediately.

Nutrition Information (Per Serving)

- Calories: 380 kcal
- Protein: 25g
- Carbohydrates: 32g
- Fiber: 6g
- Sugars: 3g (natural sugars from tomatoes)
- Fat: 18g
- Saturated Fat: 3g
- Sodium: 320mg

Cooking Time

- **Preparation Time: 10 minutes**
- **Cooking Time: 10 minutes**
- **Total Time: 20 minutes**

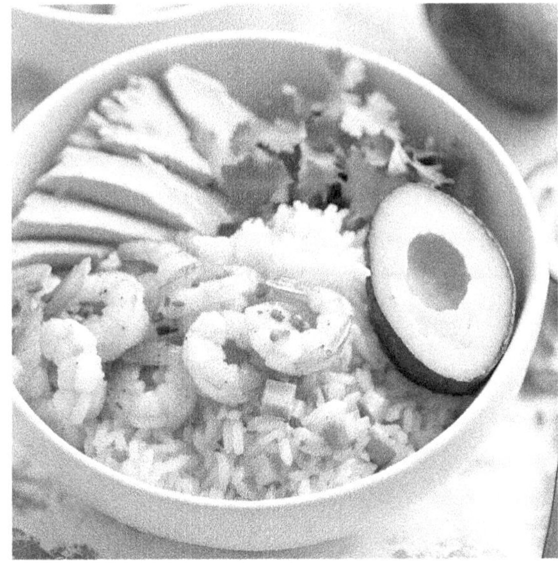

28. Tuna and Chickpea Salad

Ingredients (Serves 4)

- 2 cans (5 ounces each) tuna packed in water, drained
- 1 can (15 ounces) chickpeas, rinsed and drained
- 1/4 cup red onion, finely chopped
- 1/2 cup cherry tomatoes, halved
- 1/4 cup fresh parsley, chopped
- 2 tablespoons extra virgin olive oil
- 2 tablespoons fresh lemon juice
- 1/4 teaspoon ground black pepper

Instructions

1. Combine Ingredients: In a large bowl, combine the drained tuna, chickpeas, red onion, cherry tomatoes, and parsley.
2. Mix Dressing: In a small bowl, whisk together the olive oil, lemon juice, and black pepper.
3. Toss Salad: Pour the dressing over the salad and toss gently to combine.
4. Serve: Divide into four servings and serve immediately.

Nutrition Information (Per Serving)

- Calories: 300 kcal
- Protein: 23g
- Carbohydrates: 24g
- Fiber: 7g
- Sugars: 3g (natural sugars from chickpeas and tomatoes)
- Fat: 14g
- Saturated Fat: 2g
- Sodium: 320mg

Cooking Time

- **Preparation Time: 10 minutes**
- **Total Time: 10 minutes**

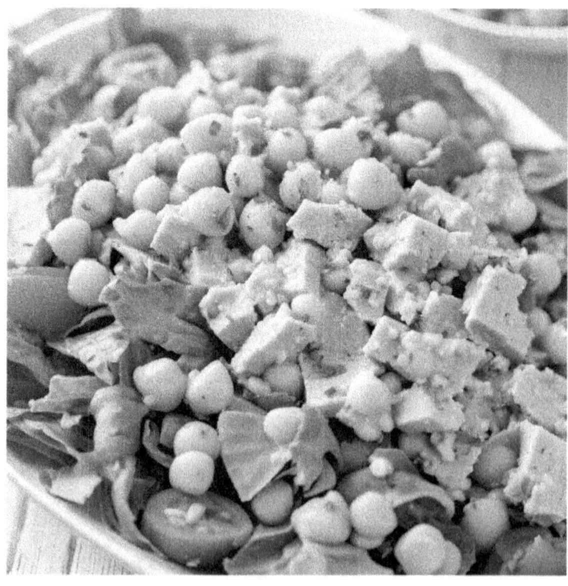

29. Broiled Sardines with Lemon and Herbs

Ingredients (Serves 4)

- 8 fresh sardines, cleaned and gutted
- 2 tablespoons extra virgin olive oil
- 2 tablespoons fresh lemon juice
- 1 tablespoon lemon zest
- 1 teaspoon dried oregano
- 1/4 teaspoon ground black pepper
- Fresh parsley for garnish (optional)
- Lemon wedges for serving (optional)

Instructions

1. Preheat Broiler: Preheat your oven's broiler to high. Line a broiler pan with aluminum foil.
2. Prepare Sardines: Place the sardines on the broiler pan. Drizzle with olive oil and lemon juice. Sprinkle with lemon zest, dried oregano, and black pepper.
3. Broil Sardines: Broil for 4-5 minutes on each side, or until the sardines are cooked through and slightly crispy on the edges.
4. Serve: Garnish with fresh parsley and serve with lemon wedges if desired. Serve warm.

Nutrition Information (Per Serving)

- Calories: 240 kcal
- Protein: 24g
- Carbohydrates: 2g
- Fiber: 1g
- Sugars: 0g
- Fat: 16g
- Saturated Fat: 3g
- Sodium: 300mg

Cooking Time

- **Preparation Time: 10 minutes**
- **Cooking Time: 10 minutes**
- **Total Time: 20 minutes**

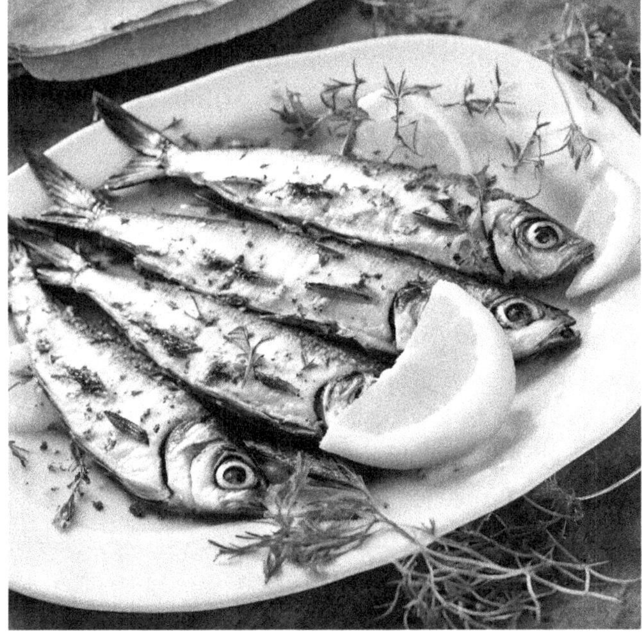

30. Grilled Swordfish with Pineapple Salsa

Ingredients (Serves 4)

- 4 swordfish steaks (about 6 ounces each)
- 2 tablespoons extra virgin olive oil
- 1 tablespoon fresh lime juice
- 1 teaspoon ground cumin
- 1/4 teaspoon ground black pepper

Pineapple Salsa:

- 1 cup fresh pineapple, diced
- 1/2 red bell pepper, diced
- 1/4 cup red onion, finely chopped
- 1 jalapeño, seeded and finely chopped
- 2 tablespoons fresh cilantro, chopped
- 1 tablespoon fresh lime juice

Instructions

1. Prepare Marinade: In a small bowl, whisk together the olive oil, lime juice, ground cumin, and black pepper.
2. Marinate Swordfish: Brush the swordfish steaks with the marinade and let sit for 10 minutes.
3. Prepare Salsa: In a medium bowl, combine the diced pineapple, red bell pepper, red onion, jalapeño, cilantro, and lime juice. Mix well and set aside.
4. Preheat Grill: Preheat your grill or grill pan to medium-high heat.
5. Grill Swordfish: Grill the swordfish steaks for about 4-5 minutes on each side, or until they are opaque and have grill marks.
6. Serve: Top the grilled swordfish with the pineapple salsa and serve warm.

Nutrition Information (Per Serving)

- Calories: 320 kcal
- Protein: 34g
- Carbohydrates: 12g
- Fiber: 2g
- Sugars: 8g (natural sugars from pineapple)
- Fat: 16g
- Saturated Fat: 3g
- Sodium: 200mg

Cooking Time

- **Preparation Time: 15 minutes**
- **Cooking Time: 10 minutes**
- **Total Time: 25 minutes**

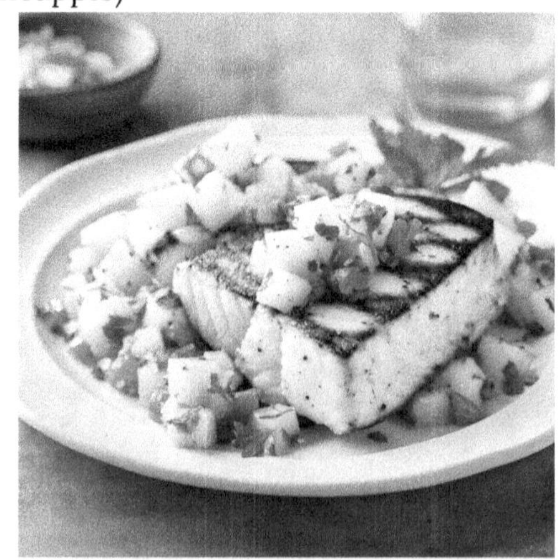

Vegetables

1. Mediterranean Quinoa Salad
Ingredients (Serves 4)
- 1 cup quinoa, rinsed
- 2 cups water or low-sodium vegetable broth
- 1 cup cherry tomatoes, halved
- 1 cucumber, diced
- 1/4 cup red onion, finely chopped
- 1/4 cup Kalamata olives, pitted and halved
- 1/4 cup feta cheese, crumbled (optional)
- 1/4 cup fresh parsley, chopped
- 1/4 cup fresh mint, chopped
- 3 tablespoons extra virgin olive oil
- 2 tablespoons fresh lemon juice
- 1 teaspoon dried oregano
- 1/4 teaspoon ground black pepper

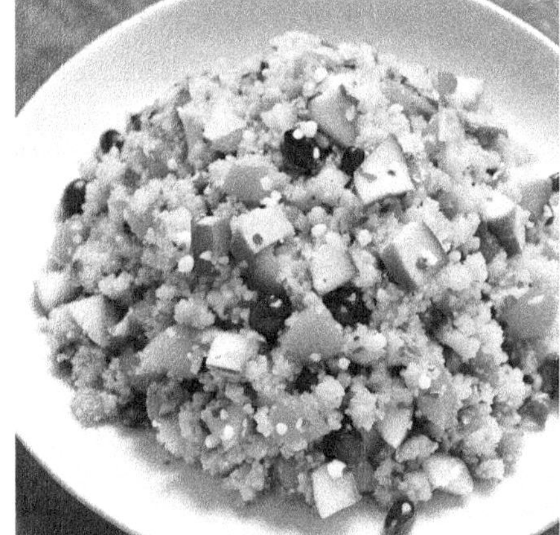

Instructions
1. Cook Quinoa: In a medium saucepan, bring the quinoa and water (or vegetable broth) to a boil. Reduce the heat to low, cover, and simmer for about 15 minutes, or until the quinoa is tender and the liquid is absorbed. Fluff with a fork and let cool.
2. Prepare Vegetables: In a large bowl, combine the cherry tomatoes, cucumber, red onion, Kalamata olives, feta cheese (if using), parsley, and mint.
3. Mix Dressing: In a small bowl, whisk together the olive oil, lemon juice, dried oregano, and black pepper.
4. Combine Salad: Add the cooked quinoa to the bowl with the vegetables. Pour the dressing over the salad and toss gently to combine.
5. Serve: Divide into four servings and serve immediately or chill for later.

Nutrition Information (Per Serving)
- Calories: 260 kcal   Protein: 6g   Carbohydrates: 30g   Fiber: 5g
- Sugars: 4g (natural sugars from vegetables)
- Fat: 14g
- Saturated Fat: 2g
- Sodium: 280mg

Cooking Time
- **Preparation Time: 10 minutes**
- **Cooking Time: 15 minutes**
- **Total Time: 25 minutes**

2. Thai Green Curry with Vegetables

Ingredients (Serves 4)

- 1 tablespoon extra virgin olive oil
- 1 onion, thinly sliced
- 2 cloves garlic, minced
- 1 tablespoon fresh ginger, grated
- 2 tablespoons green curry paste
- 1 can (14 ounces) coconut milk (light or full-fat)
- 1 cup vegetable broth (low-sodium)
- 2 cups broccoli florets
- 1 red bell pepper, thinly sliced
- 1 zucchini, sliced into half-moons
- 1 cup snap peas
- 1/4 cup fresh basil leaves, chopped
- 1/4 cup fresh cilantro, chopped
- 2 tablespoons fresh lime juice
- 1 tablespoon soy sauce (low-sodium)
- Cooked brown rice or quinoa for serving

Instructions

1. Heat Oil: In a large skillet or wok, heat the olive oil over medium heat. Add the onion and cook for about 5 minutes until softened.
2. Add Aromatics: Stir in the garlic and ginger, and cook for 1 minute until fragrant.
3. Add Curry Paste: Add the green curry paste and cook for another minute, stirring to combine with the aromatics.
4. Add Coconut Milk and Broth: Pour in the coconut milk and vegetable broth, stirring to combine. Bring to a simmer.
5. Cook Vegetables: Add the broccoli, bell pepper, zucchini, and snap peas to the skillet. Simmer for about 10 minutes until the vegetables are tender.
6. Finish with Herbs and Lime: Stir in the basil, cilantro, lime juice, and soy sauce.
7. Serve: Serve the curry over cooked brown rice or quinoa.

Nutrition Information (Per Serving)

- Calories: 300 kcal   Protein: 7g   Carbohydrates: 20g   Fiber: 6g
- Sugars: 8g (natural sugars from vegetables)   Fat: 22g   Saturated Fat: 16g   Sodium: 420mg

Cooking Time

- **Preparation Time: 10 minutes**
- **Cooking Time: 20 minutes**
- **Total Time: 30 minutes**

3. Moroccan Carrot Salad

Ingredients (Serves 4)

- 1 pound carrots, peeled and grated or thinly sliced
- 1/4 cup raisins
- 1/4 cup chopped fresh cilantro
- 1/4 cup chopped fresh mint
- 1/4 cup sliced almonds, toasted
- 2 tablespoons extra virgin olive oil
- 2 tablespoons fresh lemon juice
- 1 tablespoon honey or agave syrup
- 1 teaspoon ground cumin
- 1/4 teaspoon ground cinnamon
- 1/4 teaspoon ground black pepper

Instructions

1. Prepare Carrots: Place the grated or sliced carrots in a large bowl.
2. Add Mix-ins: Add the raisins, chopped cilantro, chopped mint, and toasted almonds to the bowl with the carrots.
3. Mix Dressing: In a small bowl, whisk together the olive oil, lemon juice, honey, ground cumin, ground cinnamon, and black pepper.
4. Combine Salad: Pour the dressing over the carrot mixture and toss well to combine.
5. Serve: Divide into four servings and serve immediately or refrigerate for up to 1 hour before serving to allow the flavors to meld.

Nutrition Information (Per Serving)

- Calories: 180 kcal
- Protein: 2g
- Carbohydrates: 21g
- Fiber: 5g
- Sugars: 12g (including natural sugars from carrots and raisins)
- Fat: 10g
- Saturated Fat: 1g
- Sodium: 50mg

Cooking Time

- **Preparation Time: 10 minutes**
- **Total Time: 10 minutes**

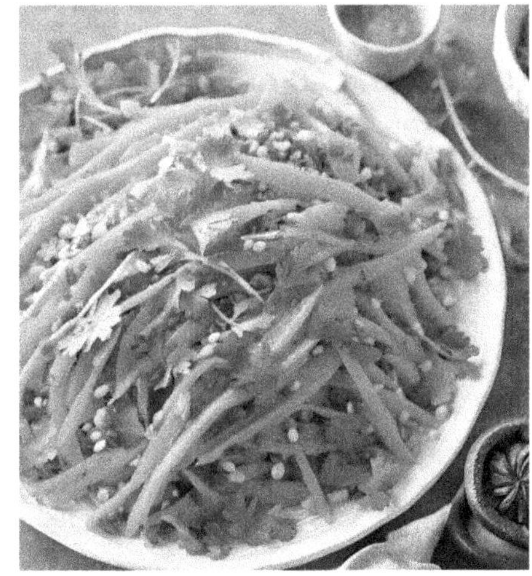

4. Indian Spiced Cauliflower

Ingredients (Serves 4)

- 1 large head cauliflower, cut into florets
- 2 tablespoons extra virgin olive oil
- 1 tablespoon curry powder
- 1 teaspoon ground turmeric
- 1 teaspoon ground cumin
- 1 teaspoon ground coriander
- 1/4 teaspoon ground black pepper
- 1/4 cup fresh cilantro, chopped
- Lemon wedges for serving (optional)

Instructions

1. Preheat Oven: Preheat your oven to 400°F (200°C). Line a baking sheet with parchment paper.
2. Prepare Cauliflower: In a large bowl, toss the cauliflower florets with olive oil, curry powder, turmeric, cumin, coriander, and black pepper until well coated.
3. Roast Cauliflower: Spread the cauliflower in a single layer on the prepared baking sheet. Roast in the preheated oven for 25-30 minutes, or until the cauliflower is tender and golden brown, stirring halfway through.
4. Garnish and Serve: Remove from the oven and sprinkle with fresh cilantro. Serve with lemon wedges if desired.

Nutrition Information (Per Serving)

- Calories: 120 kcal
- Protein: 3g
- Carbohydrates: 10g
- Fiber: 4g
- Sugars: 3g (natural sugars from cauliflower)
- Fat: 8g
- Saturated Fat: 1g
- Sodium: 55mg

Cooking Time

- **Preparation Time: 10 minutes**
- **Cooking Time: 30 minutes**
- **Total Time: 40 minutes**

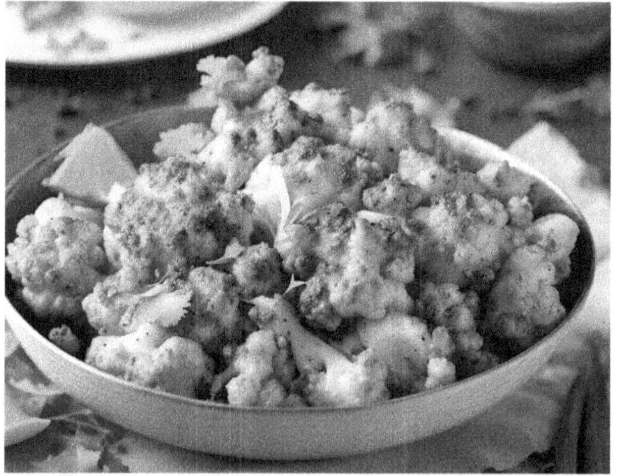

5. Chinese Stir-Fried Bok Choy

Ingredients (Serves 4)

- 1 pound baby bok choy, trimmed and washed
- 2 tablespoons extra virgin olive oil
- 3 cloves garlic, minced
- 1 tablespoon fresh ginger, grated
- 2 tablespoons low-sodium soy sauce
- 1 tablespoon rice vinegar
- 1 tablespoon sesame oil
- 1/4 teaspoon ground black pepper
- 1 tablespoon sesame seeds for garnish (optional)

Instructions

1. Prepare Bok Choy: Slice the bok choy in half lengthwise if large, leaving smaller ones whole.
2. Heat Oil: In a large skillet or wok, heat the olive oil over medium-high heat. Add the minced garlic and grated ginger, and cook for about 1 minute until fragrant.
3. Stir-Fry Bok Choy: Add the bok choy to the skillet and stir-fry for 3-4 minutes until the greens are wilted and the stems are tender.
4. Add Sauce: Stir in the soy sauce, rice vinegar, sesame oil, and black pepper. Cook for another 1-2 minutes until heated through.
5. Serve: Transfer to a serving dish and garnish with sesame seeds if desired. Serve immediately.

Nutrition Information (Per Serving)

- Calories: 110 kcal
- Protein: 3g
- Carbohydrates: 8g
- Fiber: 3g
- Sugars: 3g (natural sugars from bok choy)
- Fat: 8g
- Saturated Fat: 1g
- Sodium: 320mg

Cooking Time

- **Preparation Time: 5 minutes**
- **Cooking Time: 10 minutes**
- **Total Time: 15 minutes**

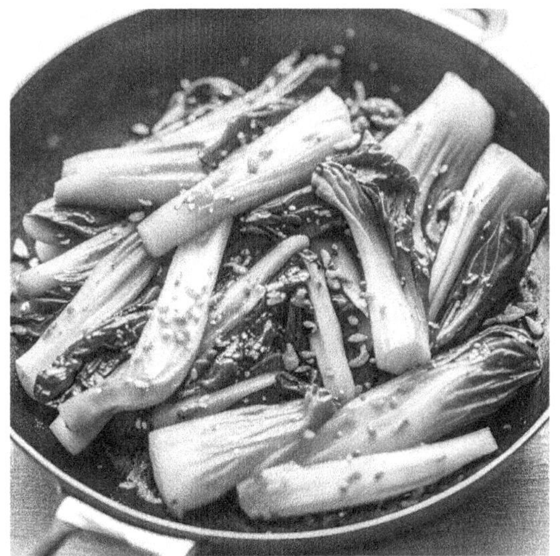

6. Italian Caponata

Ingredients (Serves 4)

- 1 large eggplant, diced
- 1 red bell pepper, diced
- 1 yellow bell pepper, diced
- 1 medium onion, chopped
- 3 cloves garlic, minced
- 2 celery stalks, chopped
- 3 tablespoons extra virgin olive oil
- 1/4 cup green olives, pitted and chopped
- 2 tablespoons capers, drained
- 1/4 cup tomato paste
- 1/4 cup red wine vinegar
- 1 tablespoon honey or agave syrup
- 1/4 teaspoon ground black pepper
- 1/4 cup fresh basil, chopped

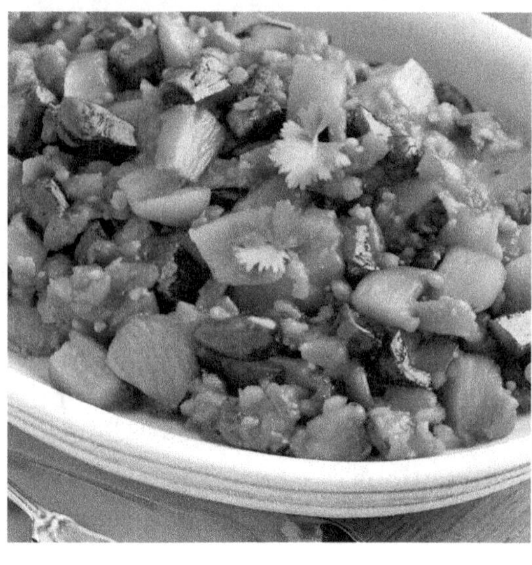

Instructions

1. Prepare Eggplant: Sprinkle the diced eggplant with a pinch of salt and let it sit in a colander for 30 minutes to draw out moisture. Rinse and pat dry with paper towels.
2. Sauté Vegetables: In a large skillet, heat the olive oil over medium heat. Add the onion and celery, and cook until softened, about 5 minutes.
3. Add Eggplant and Peppers: Stir in the eggplant, red bell pepper, yellow bell pepper, and garlic. Cook for another 10 minutes until the vegetables are tender.
4. Add Remaining Ingredients: Add the tomato paste, red wine vinegar, honey, chopped olives, capers, and black pepper. Stir to combine.
5. Simmer: Reduce the heat and let the mixture simmer for 15-20 minutes, stirring occasionally, until the flavors meld together.
6. Finish and Serve: Stir in the fresh basil just before serving. Serve warm or at room temperature.

Nutrition Information (Per Serving)

- Calories: 180 kcal Protein: 3g Carbohydrates: 25g Fiber: 7g
- Sugars: 12g (including natural sugars from vegetables and honey)
- Fat: 8g Saturated Fat: 1g Sodium: 320mg

Cooking Time

- **Preparation Time: 10 minutes**
- **Cooking Time: 35 minutes**
- **Total Time: 45 minutes**

7. Mexican Grilled Vegetable Tacos

Ingredients (Serves 4)

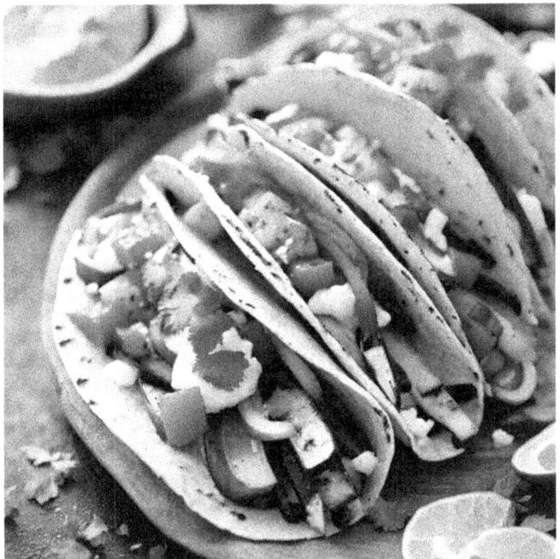

- 2 zucchini, sliced into rounds
- 1 red bell pepper, sliced into strips
- 1 yellow bell pepper, sliced into strips
- 1 red onion, sliced into rings
- 2 tablespoons extra virgin olive oil
- 1 teaspoon ground cumin
- 1 teaspoon smoked paprika
- 1/4 teaspoon ground black pepper
- 8 small corn tortillas
- 1/2 cup fresh cilantro, chopped
- 1/2 cup crumbled feta cheese (optional)
- Lime wedges for serving

Instructions

1. Preheat Grill: Preheat your grill or grill pan to medium-high heat.
2. Prepare Vegetables: In a large bowl, toss the zucchini, bell peppers, and red onion with olive oil, ground cumin, smoked paprika, and black pepper.
3. Grill Vegetables: Place the vegetables on the grill and cook for about 5-7 minutes, turning occasionally, until they are tender and have grill marks.
4. Warm Tortillas: While the vegetables are grilling, warm the corn tortillas on the grill for about 1 minute on each side.
5. Assemble Tacos: Fill each tortilla with the grilled vegetables. Top with chopped cilantro and crumbled feta cheese if using.
6. Serve: Serve the tacos with lime wedges on the side.

Nutrition Information (Per Serving)

- Calories: 230 kcal
- Protein: 5g
- Carbohydrates: 30g
- Fiber: 6g
- Sugars: 6g (natural sugars from vegetables)
- Fat: 11g
- Saturated Fat: 2g
- Sodium: 140mg

Cooking Time

- **Preparation Time: 10 minutes**
- **Cooking Time: 15 minutes**
- **Total Time: 25 minutes**

8. Lebanese Tabbouleh
Ingredients (Serves 4)

- 1/2 cup bulgur wheat
- 1 cup boiling water
- 2 cups fresh parsley, finely chopped
- 1/2 cup fresh mint, finely chopped
- 1/4 cup green onions, finely chopped
- 2 large tomatoes, diced
- 1 cucumber, diced
- 1/4 cup extra virgin olive oil
- 3 tablespoons fresh lemon juice
- 1/4 teaspoon ground black pepper

Instructions

1. Prepare Bulgur: Place the bulgur wheat in a large bowl and pour the boiling water over it. Cover and let sit for about 20 minutes, or until the bulgur is tender. Drain any excess water.
2. Combine Vegetables and Herbs: In a large bowl, combine the parsley, mint, green onions, tomatoes, and cucumber.
3. Mix Dressing: In a small bowl, whisk together the olive oil, lemon juice, and black pepper.
4. Assemble Salad: Add the bulgur wheat to the bowl with the vegetables. Pour the dressing over the salad and toss to combine.
5. Serve: Divide into four servings and serve immediately or refrigerate for later.

Nutrition Information (Per Serving)

- Calories: 180 kcal
- Protein: 3g
- Carbohydrates: 21g
- Fiber: 7g
- Sugars: 5g (natural sugars from vegetables)
- Fat: 10g
- Saturated Fat: 1g
- Sodium: 30mg

Cooking Time

- **Preparation Time: 15 minutes**
- **Total Time: 15 minutes (plus 20 minutes for bulgur soaking)**

9. Korean Bibimbap with Vegetables

Ingredients (Serves 4)

- 2 cups cooked brown rice
- 1 cup spinach, blanched
- 1 cup carrot, julienned
- 1 cup zucchini, julienned
- 1 cup mushrooms, sliced
- 1/4 cup bean sprouts
- 4 eggs (optional)
- 2 tablespoons extra virgin olive oil
- 2 tablespoons soy sauce (low-sodium)
- 1 tablespoon sesame oil
- 1 tablespoon gochujang (Korean red chili paste)
- 1 teaspoon sesame seeds for garnish

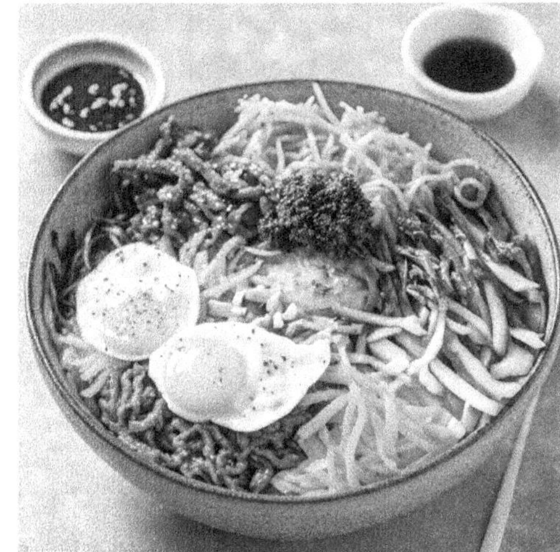

Instructions

1. Prepare Vegetables: Heat 1 tablespoon of olive oil in a large skillet over medium heat. Add the carrots, zucchini, mushrooms, and bean sprouts, and sauté for 3-4 minutes until tender. Remove from the skillet and set aside.
2. Cook Spinach: In the same skillet, add the blanched spinach and stir in the soy sauce. Cook for 1 minute until the spinach is well coated.
3. Fry Eggs: In a separate skillet, heat the remaining tablespoon of olive oil and fry the eggs to your desired doneness, if using.
4. Assemble Bibimbap: Divide the cooked brown rice into four bowls. Arrange the cooked vegetables and spinach on top of the rice. Add a fried egg to each bowl if using.
5. Add Toppings: Drizzle each bowl with sesame oil and a dollop of gochujang. Sprinkle with sesame seeds.
6. Serve: Serve immediately, mixing the ingredients together before eating.

Nutrition Information (Per Serving without Egg)

- Calories: 280 kcal   Protein: 6g Carbohydrates: 38g   Fiber: 6g
- Sugars: 5g (natural sugars from vegetables)
- Fat: 11g
- Saturated Fat: 1g
- Sodium: 320mg

Cooking Time

- **Preparation Time: 10 minutes**
- **Cooking Time: 10 minutes**
- **Total Time: 20 minutes**

10. Vietnamese Fresh Spring Rolls
Ingredients (Serves 4, makes 8 rolls)

- 8 rice paper wrappers
- 1 cup cooked rice noodles
- 1 cup shredded lettuce
- 1/2 cup carrots, julienned
- 1/2 cup cucumber, julienned
- 1/2 cup fresh mint leaves
- 1/2 cup fresh cilantro leaves
- 1/4 cup fresh basil leaves
- 8 shrimp, cooked and halved lengthwise (optional)
- 1/4 cup peanut sauce or hoisin sauce for dipping

Instructions

1. Prepare Ingredients: Arrange the rice noodles, lettuce, carrots, cucumber, mint, cilantro, basil, and shrimp (if using) on a work surface.
2. Soften Rice Paper: Fill a large bowl with warm water. Dip one rice paper wrapper into the water for about 10-15 seconds until it becomes soft and pliable.
3. Assemble Rolls: Lay the softened rice paper on a flat surface. Place a small amount of rice noodles, lettuce, carrots, cucumber, mint, cilantro, basil, and shrimp (if using) near the bottom of the wrapper.
4. Roll: Fold the bottom of the wrapper over the filling, fold in the sides, and roll up tightly. Repeat with the remaining wrappers and fillings.
5. Serve: Serve the spring rolls with peanut sauce or hoisin sauce for dipping.

Nutrition Information (Per Serving without Shrimp)

- Calories: 160 kcal
- Protein: 3g
- Carbohydrates: 32g
- Fiber: 3g
- Sugars: 2g (natural sugars from vegetables)
- Fat: 2g
- Saturated Fat: 0g
- Sodium: 50mg

Cooking Time

- **Preparation Time: 20 minutes**
- **Total Time: 20 minutes**

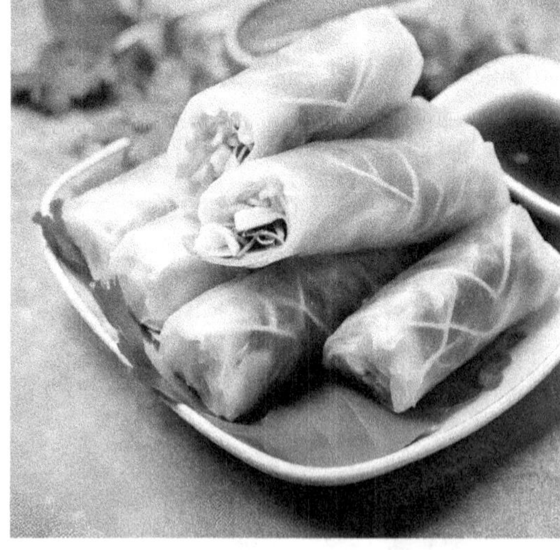

11. Turkish Eggplant (Imam Bayildi)

Ingredients (Serves 4)

- 2 large eggplants, halved lengthwise
- 1/4 cup extra virgin olive oil
- 1 onion, finely chopped
- 3 cloves garlic, minced
- 2 tomatoes, diced
- 1 green bell pepper, diced
- 1 tablespoon tomato paste
- 1 teaspoon ground cumin
- 1 teaspoon ground coriander
- 1/4 teaspoon ground black pepper
- 1/4 cup fresh parsley, chopped
- Lemon wedges for serving (optional)

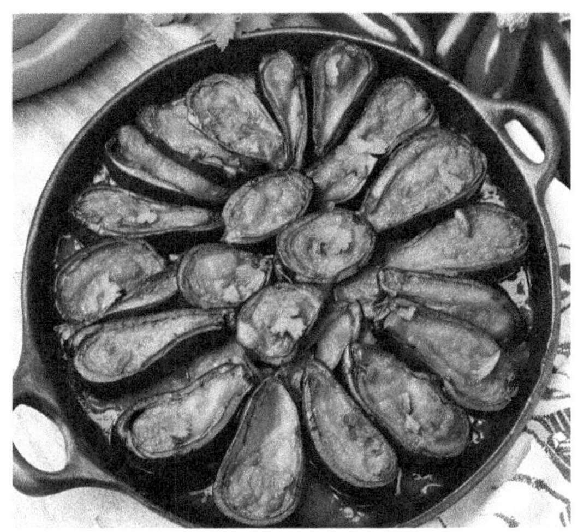

Instructions

1. Preheat Oven: Preheat your oven to 375°F (190°C). Line a baking dish with parchment paper.
2. Prepare Eggplants: Brush the cut sides of the eggplants with olive oil and place them cut-side down on the baking dish. Roast in the preheated oven for 20 minutes until tender.
3. Sauté Filling: While the eggplants are roasting, heat the remaining olive oil in a skillet over medium heat. Add the onion and garlic, and cook until softened, about 5 minutes. Stir in the tomatoes, bell pepper, tomato paste, cumin, coriander, and black pepper. Cook for another 10 minutes until the mixture is thickened.
4. Stuff Eggplants: Remove the eggplants from the oven and carefully scoop out some of the flesh to make a cavity. Fill each eggplant half with the vegetable mixture.
5. Bake: Return the stuffed eggplants to the oven and bake for an additional 15 minutes.
6. Serve: Garnish with fresh parsley and serve warm with lemon wedges if desired.

Nutrition Information (Per Serving)

- Calories: 220 kcal Protein: 3g Carbohydrates: 20g Fiber: 7g
- Sugars: 10g (natural sugars from vegetables)
- Fat: 14g Saturated Fat: 2g Sodium: 180mg

Cooking Time

- **Preparation Time: 10 minutes**
- **Cooking Time: 35 minutes**
- **Total Time: 45 minutes**

12. Ethiopian Lentil Stew (Misir Wot)

Ingredients (Serves 4)

- 1 cup red lentils, rinsed
- 2 tablespoons extra virgin olive oil
- 1 onion, finely chopped
- 3 cloves garlic, minced
- 1 tablespoon fresh ginger, grated
- 1 tablespoon berbere spice mix
- 1/2 teaspoon ground cumin
- 2 cups low-sodium vegetable broth
- 1 cup diced tomatoes (canned, no salt added)
- 1/4 cup fresh cilantro, chopped

Instructions

1. Cook Aromatics: In a large pot, heat the olive oil over medium heat. Add the onion and cook until softened, about 5 minutes. Stir in the garlic and ginger, and cook for another minute.
2. Add Spices: Add the berbere spice mix and ground cumin, and cook for 1-2 minutes until fragrant.
3. Cook Lentils: Stir in the lentils, vegetable broth, and diced tomatoes. Bring to a simmer.
4. Simmer: Reduce the heat to low, cover, and simmer for about 20-25 minutes until the lentils are tender and the stew is thickened.
5. Serve: Stir in the fresh cilantro and serve warm.

Nutrition Information (Per Serving)

- Calories: 240 kcal
- Protein: 12g
- Carbohydrates: 34g
- Fiber: 10g
- Sugars: 8g (natural sugars from tomatoes)
- Fat: 8g
- Saturated Fat: 1g
- Sodium: 220mg

Cooking Time

- **Preparation Time: 10 minutes**
- **Cooking Time: 25 minutes**
- **Total Time: 35 minutes**

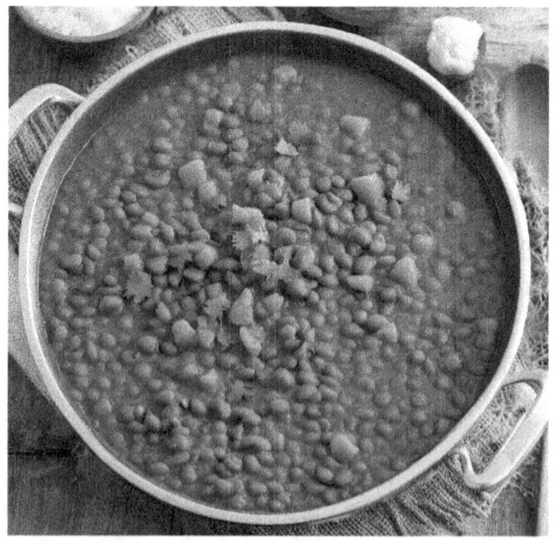

13. Middle Eastern Roasted Vegetables

Ingredients (Serves 4)

- 1 large eggplant, diced
- 1 red bell pepper, sliced
- 1 yellow bell pepper, sliced
- 1 zucchini, sliced into rounds
- 1 red onion, sliced
- 2 tablespoons extra virgin olive oil
- 1 teaspoon ground cumin
- 1 teaspoon ground coriander
- 1 teaspoon ground turmeric
- 1/4 teaspoon ground black pepper
- 1/4 cup fresh parsley, chopped
- 2 tablespoons tahini
- 2 tablespoons fresh lemon juice
- 1 tablespoon water
- 1/4 teaspoon garlic powder

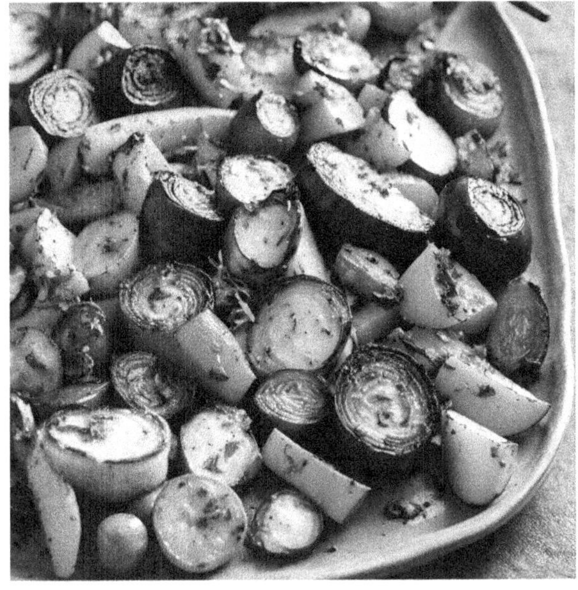

Instructions

1. Preheat Oven: Preheat your oven to 400°F (200°C). Line a baking sheet with parchment paper.
2. Prepare Vegetables: Place the eggplant, bell peppers, zucchini, and red onion in a large bowl. Drizzle with olive oil and sprinkle with cumin, coriander, turmeric, and black pepper. Toss to coat evenly.
3. Roast Vegetables: Spread the vegetables in a single layer on the prepared baking sheet. Roast in the preheated oven for 25-30 minutes, or until tender and lightly browned.
4. Prepare Tahini Sauce: While the vegetables are roasting, mix the tahini, lemon juice, water, and garlic powder in a small bowl until smooth.
5. Serve: Transfer the roasted vegetables to a serving platter. Drizzle with the tahini sauce and garnish with fresh parsley. Serve warm.

Nutrition Information (Per Serving)

- Calories: 180 kcal
- Protein: 4g
- Carbohydrates: 20g
- Fiber: 6g
- Sugars: 8g (natural sugars from vegetables)
- Fat: 10g
- Saturated Fat: 1g
- Sodium: 40mg

Cooking Time

- **Preparation Time: 10 minutes**
- **Cooking Time: 30 minutes**
- **Total Time: 40 minutes**

14. Caribbean Callaloo

Ingredients (Serves 4)

- 1 pound fresh callaloo leaves (or substitute with spinach or Swiss chard), washed and chopped
- 2 tablespoons extra virgin olive oil
- 1 onion, chopped
- 2 cloves garlic, minced
- 1 bell pepper (any color), chopped
- 1 cup diced tomatoes (canned or fresh)
- 1/4 teaspoon ground black pepper
- 1/2 teaspoon thyme leaves
- 1/4 teaspoon allspice
- 1/4 cup coconut milk

Instructions

1. Heat Oil: In a large pot, heat the olive oil over medium heat. Add the onion and garlic and sauté for 2-3 minutes until softened.
2. Add Bell Pepper and Tomatoes: Stir in the chopped bell pepper and diced tomatoes. Cook for another 5 minutes until the tomatoes start to break down.
3. Add Callaloo: Add the chopped callaloo leaves, black pepper, thyme, and allspice. Stir well to combine.
4. Cook Down: Cover and cook for about 10-15 minutes until the callaloo is tender.
5. Add Coconut Milk: Stir in the coconut milk and cook for an additional 2-3 minutes.
6. Serve: Serve warm as a side dish or over rice.

Nutrition Information (Per Serving)

- Calories: 150 kcal
- Protein: 3g
- Carbohydrates: 12g
- Fiber: 5g
- Sugars: 4g (natural sugars from vegetables)
- Fat: 10g
- Saturated Fat: 5g
- Sodium: 50mg

Cooking Time

- **Preparation Time: 10 minutes**
- **Cooking Time: 20 minutes**
- **Total Time: 30 minutes**

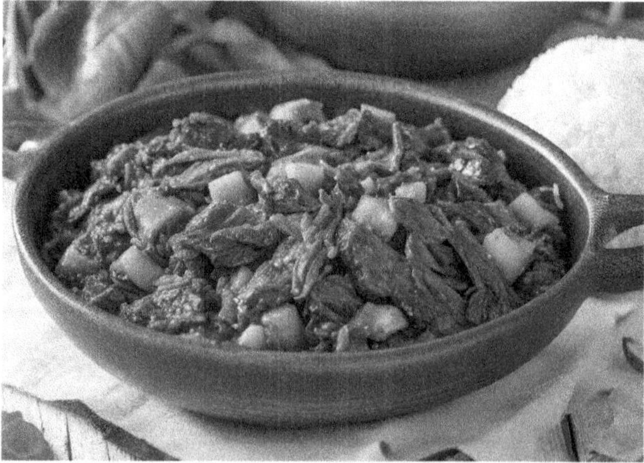

15. Argentinian Chimichurri Vegetables

Ingredients (Serves 4)

- 2 cups broccoli florets
- 2 cups cauliflower florets
- 2 bell peppers (red and yellow), sliced
- 1 zucchini, sliced into rounds
- 2 tablespoons extra virgin olive oil
- 1/4 teaspoon ground black pepper

Chimichurri Sauce:

- 1/2 cup fresh parsley, chopped
- 1/4 cup fresh cilantro, chopped
- 1/4 cup red wine vinegar
- 3 tablespoons extra virgin olive oil
- 3 cloves garlic, minced
- 1 teaspoon dried oregano
- 1/4 teaspoon red pepper flakes
- 1/4 teaspoon ground black pepper

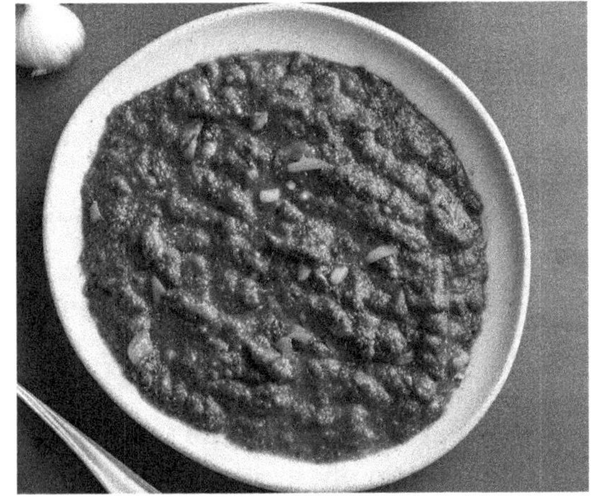

Instructions

1. Preheat Oven: Preheat your oven to 400°F (200°C). Line a baking sheet with parchment paper.
2. Prepare Vegetables: Place the broccoli, cauliflower, bell peppers, and zucchini in a large bowl. Drizzle with olive oil and sprinkle with black pepper. Toss to coat evenly.
3. Roast Vegetables: Spread the vegetables in a single layer on the prepared baking sheet. Roast in the preheated oven for 25-30 minutes until tender and lightly browned.
4. Make Chimichurri Sauce: While the vegetables are roasting, combine the chopped parsley, cilantro, red wine vinegar, olive oil, minced garlic, oregano, red pepper flakes, and black pepper in a bowl. Mix well.
5. Serve: Transfer the roasted vegetables to a serving platter. Drizzle with the chimichurri sauce and serve warm.

Nutrition Information (Per Serving)

- Calories: 210 kcal Protein: 4g Carbohydrates: 18g Fiber: 6g
- Sugars: 7g (natural sugars from vegetables)
- Fat: 15g Saturated Fat: 2g Sodium: 40mg

Cooking Time

- **Preparation Time: 10 minutes**
- **Cooking Time: 30 minutes**
- **Total Time: 40 minutes**

16. Greek Briam (Roasted Vegetables)

Ingredients (Serves 4)

- 2 potatoes, thinly sliced
- 2 zucchinis, thinly sliced
- 1 eggplant, diced
- 2 tomatoes, sliced
- 1 red onion, thinly sliced
- 3 cloves garlic, minced
- 1/4 cup extra virgin olive oil
- 2 tablespoons fresh parsley, chopped
- 1 teaspoon dried oregano
- 1/4 teaspoon ground black pepper
- 1/4 cup crumbled feta cheese (optional)

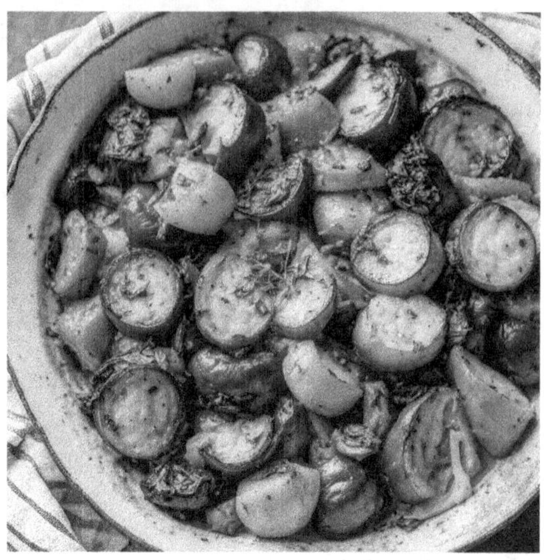

Instructions

1. Preheat Oven: Preheat your oven to 375°F (190°C). Grease a large baking dish with a little olive oil.
2. Layer Vegetables: Arrange the potatoes, zucchinis, eggplant, tomatoes, and red onion in the baking dish, layering them in a pattern if desired. Sprinkle the minced garlic over the top.
3. Season and Drizzle: Drizzle with the olive oil and sprinkle with parsley, oregano, and black pepper.
4. Bake: Cover with aluminum foil and bake in the preheated oven for 30 minutes. Remove the foil and bake for an additional 15 minutes until the vegetables are tender and slightly browned.
5. Serve: Garnish with crumbled feta cheese if desired and serve warm.

Nutrition Information (Per Serving)

- Calories: 240 kcal
- Protein: 4g
- Carbohydrates: 30g
- Fiber: 8g
- Sugars: 9g (natural sugars from vegetables)
- Fat: 12g
- Saturated Fat: 2g
- Sodium: 70mg

Cooking Time

- **Preparation Time: 10 minutes**
- **Cooking Time: 45 minutes**
- **Total Time: 55 minutes**

17. Moroccan Zaalouk (Eggplant Dip)

Ingredients (Serves 4)

- 2 large eggplants, peeled and diced
- 2 tomatoes, diced
- 3 cloves garlic, minced
- 2 tablespoons extra virgin olive oil
- 1 teaspoon ground cumin
- 1 teaspoon smoked paprika
- 1/4 teaspoon ground black pepper
- 1/4 teaspoon ground coriander
- 1/4 cup fresh parsley, chopped
- 1/4 cup fresh cilantro, chopped
- 2 tablespoons fresh lemon juice

Instructions

1. Cook Eggplant: In a large pot, heat the olive oil over medium heat. Add the diced eggplant and cook for about 10 minutes until softened.
2. Add Tomatoes and Garlic: Stir in the diced tomatoes and minced garlic. Cook for another 5 minutes until the tomatoes begin to break down.
3. Add Spices: Add the cumin, smoked paprika, black pepper, and ground coriander. Stir well to combine.
4. Simmer: Reduce the heat to low and simmer for about 15 minutes, stirring occasionally, until the mixture thickens and the flavors meld.
5. Finish with Herbs and Lemon: Stir in the fresh parsley, cilantro, and lemon juice.
6. Serve: Serve warm or at room temperature as a dip with bread or as a side dish.

Nutrition Information (Per Serving)

- Calories: 140 kcal
- Protein: 2g
- Carbohydrates: 15g
- Fiber: 6g
- Sugars: 8g (natural sugars from vegetables)
- Fat: 9g
- Saturated Fat: 1g
- Sodium: 40mg

Cooking Time

- **Preparation Time: 10 minutes**
- **Cooking Time: 30 minutes**
- **Total Time: 40 minutes**

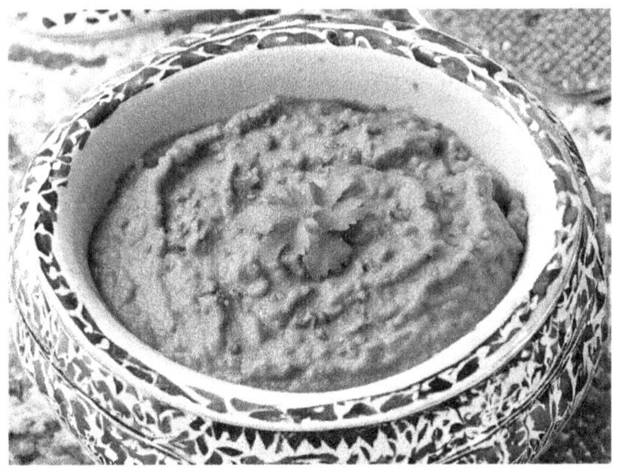

18. Peruvian Quinoa and Vegetable Stew
Ingredients (Serves 4)

- 1 cup quinoa, rinsed
- 1 tablespoon extra virgin olive oil
- 1 onion, chopped
- 3 cloves garlic, minced
- 2 carrots, diced
- 1 red bell pepper, diced
- 1 zucchini, diced
- 1 cup diced tomatoes (canned or fresh)
- 4 cups low-sodium vegetable broth
- 1 teaspoon ground cumin
- 1/2 teaspoon ground coriander
- 1/4 teaspoon ground black pepper
- 1 cup kale, chopped
- 1/4 cup fresh cilantro, chopped
- 1 tablespoon fresh lime juice

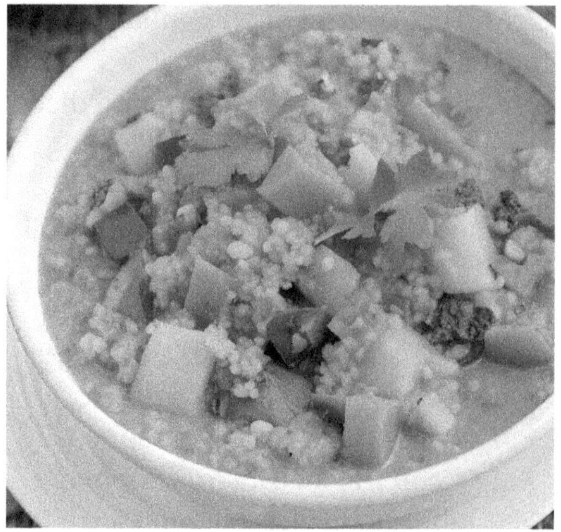

Instructions

1. Heat Oil: In a large pot, heat the olive oil over medium heat. Add the onion and garlic, and cook until softened, about 5 minutes.
2. Add Vegetables: Stir in the carrots, bell pepper, zucchini, and diced tomatoes. Cook for another 5 minutes until the vegetables begin to soften.
3. Add Quinoa and Spices: Add the rinsed quinoa, vegetable broth, cumin, coriander, and black pepper. Bring to a boil.
4. Simmer: Reduce the heat to low and simmer for about 20 minutes until the quinoa is tender and the stew has thickened.
5. Add Kale: Stir in the chopped kale and cook for an additional 5 minutes until the kale is wilted.
6. Finish with Herbs and Lime: Stir in the fresh cilantro and lime juice.
7. Serve: Serve warm.

Nutrition Information (Per Serving)

- Calories: 220 kcal Protein: 7g Carbohydrates: 32g Fiber: 8g
- Sugars: 9g (natural sugars from vegetables)
- Fat: 6g Saturated Fat: 1g Sodium: 300mg

Cooking Time

- **Preparation Time: 10 minutes**
- **Cooking Time: 30 minutes**
- **Total Time: 40 minutes**

19. Korean Spicy Stir-Fried Vegetables (Kimchi Bokkeum)

Ingredients (Serves 4)

- 1 cup kimchi, chopped
- 2 cups napa cabbage, chopped
- 1 carrot, julienned
- 1 zucchini, julienned
- 1/2 onion, sliced
- 2 tablespoons extra virgin olive oil
- 2 cloves garlic, minced
- 1 tablespoon gochujang (Korean red chili paste)
- 1 tablespoon soy sauce (low-sodium)
- 1 tablespoon sesame oil
- 1/4 teaspoon ground black pepper
- 1 tablespoon sesame seeds for garnish
- 2 green onions, chopped for garnish

Instructions

1. Heat Oil: In a large skillet or wok, heat the olive oil over medium-high heat. Add the garlic and onion, and sauté for 2-3 minutes until fragrant.
2. Add Vegetables: Add the napa cabbage, carrot, and zucchini. Stir-fry for about 5 minutes until the vegetables start to soften.
3. Add Kimchi and Seasoning: Stir in the chopped kimchi, gochujang, soy sauce, sesame oil, and black pepper. Cook for an additional 3-4 minutes until everything is well combined and heated through.
4. Garnish and Serve: Remove from heat and garnish with sesame seeds and chopped green onions. Serve immediately.

Nutrition Information (Per Serving)

- Calories: 150 kcal
- Protein: 3g
- Carbohydrates: 12g
- Fiber: 4g
- Sugars: 5g (natural sugars from vegetables)
- Fat: 10g
- Saturated Fat: 2g
- Sodium: 600mg

Cooking Time

- **Preparation Time: 10 minutes**
- **Cooking Time: 10 minutes**
- **Total Time: 20 minutes**

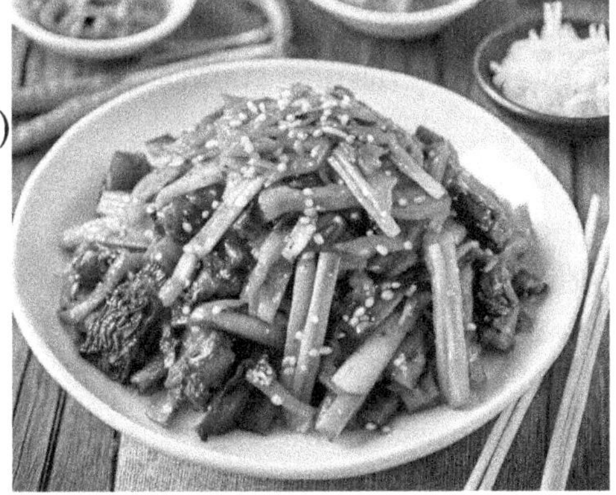

20. Italian Panzanella Salad

Ingredients (Serves 4)

- 4 cups day-old bread, cubed
- 2 cups cherry tomatoes, halved
- 1 cucumber, diced
- 1 red bell pepper, diced
- 1/2 red onion, thinly sliced
- 1/4 cup capers, drained
- 1/4 cup fresh basil leaves, chopped
- 1/4 cup extra virgin olive oil
- 2 tablespoons red wine vinegar
- 1 teaspoon dried oregano
- 1/4 teaspoon ground black pepper

Instructions

1. Toast Bread: Preheat your oven to 375°F (190°C). Spread the bread cubes on a baking sheet and toast for about 10 minutes, or until golden and slightly crisp.
2. Combine Vegetables: In a large bowl, combine the cherry tomatoes, cucumber, red bell pepper, red onion, capers, and basil.
3. Make Dressing: In a small bowl, whisk together the olive oil, red wine vinegar, dried oregano, and black pepper.
4. Assemble Salad: Add the toasted bread cubes to the bowl with the vegetables. Pour the dressing over the top and toss to combine.
5. Serve: Allow the salad to sit for about 10 minutes before serving to let the bread soak up the flavors.

Nutrition Information (Per Serving)

- Calories: 250 kcal
- Protein: 5g
- Carbohydrates: 30g
- Fiber: 5g
- Sugars: 6g (natural sugars from vegetables)
- Fat: 12g
- Saturated Fat: 2g
- Sodium: 350mg

Cooking Time

- **Preparation Time: 10 minutes**
- **Cooking Time: 10 minutes**
- **Total Time: 20 minutes**

21. Vietnamese Lemongrass Tofu with Vegetables

Ingredients (Serves 4)

- 1 block (14 ounces) firm tofu, drained and cubed
- 2 tablespoons extra virgin olive oil
- 2 stalks lemongrass, finely chopped
- 3 cloves garlic, minced
- 1 red bell pepper, sliced
- 1 carrot, julienned
- 1 zucchini, sliced into rounds
- 2 tablespoons soy sauce (low-sodium)
- 1 tablespoon fresh lime juice
- 1/4 teaspoon ground black pepper
- Fresh cilantro for garnish

Instructions

1. Marinate Tofu: In a bowl, toss the tofu cubes with 1 tablespoon of olive oil, lemongrass, and garlic. Let marinate for at least 10 minutes.
2. Cook Tofu: In a large skillet, heat the remaining tablespoon of olive oil over medium-high heat. Add the tofu and cook for about 5 minutes, turning occasionally, until golden brown on all sides.
3. Add Vegetables: Add the red bell pepper, carrot, and zucchini to the skillet. Cook for another 5 minutes until the vegetables are tender.
4. Season: Stir in the soy sauce, lime juice, and black pepper. Cook for an additional 2 minutes.
5. Serve: Garnish with fresh cilantro and serve warm.

Nutrition Information (Per Serving)

- Calories: 220 kcal
- Protein: 10g
- Carbohydrates: 12g
- Fiber: 4g
- Sugars: 4g (natural sugars from vegetables)
- Fat: 15g
- Saturated Fat: 2g
- Sodium: 400mg

Cooking Time

- **Preparation Time: 10 minutes**
- **Marinating Time: 10 minutes**
- **Cooking Time: 12 minutes**
- **Total Time: 32 minutes**

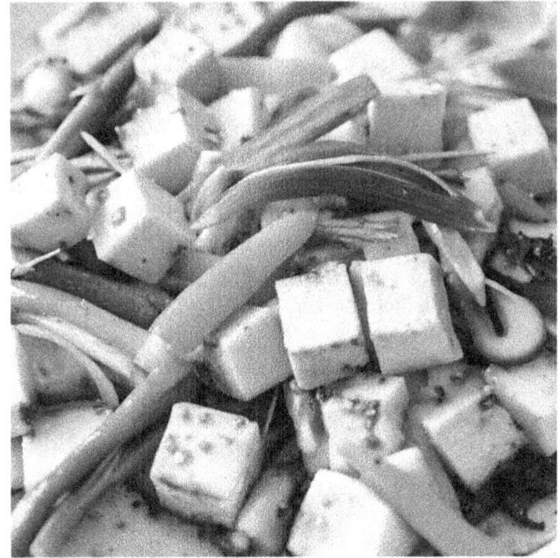

22. Ethiopian Stewed Collard Greens

Ingredients (Serves 4)

- 1 pound collard greens, stems removed and chopped
- 2 tablespoons extra virgin olive oil
- 1 onion, chopped
- 3 cloves garlic, minced
- 1 teaspoon fresh ginger, grated
- 1 cup diced tomatoes (canned or fresh)
- 1 teaspoon berbere spice mix
- 1/4 teaspoon ground black pepper
- 1/4 cup vegetable broth (low-sodium)

Instructions

1. Cook Onion and Garlic: In a large pot, heat the olive oil over medium heat. Add the onion and cook for about 5 minutes until softened. Stir in the garlic and ginger and cook for another minute.
2. Add Tomatoes and Spices: Add the diced tomatoes, berbere spice mix, and black pepper. Cook for another 5 minutes until the tomatoes start to break down.
3. Cook Collard Greens: Add the collard greens and vegetable broth. Stir well to combine. Cover and simmer for about 15 minutes until the greens are tender.
4. Serve: Serve warm as a side dish.

Nutrition Information (Per Serving)

- Calories: 120 kcal
- Protein: 2g
- Carbohydrates: 10g
- Fiber: 4g
- Sugars: 4g (natural sugars from tomatoes)
- Fat: 9g
- Saturated Fat: 1g
- Sodium: 150mg

Cooking Time

- **Preparation Time: 10 minutes**
- **Cooking Time: 25 minutes**
- **Total Time: 35 minutes**

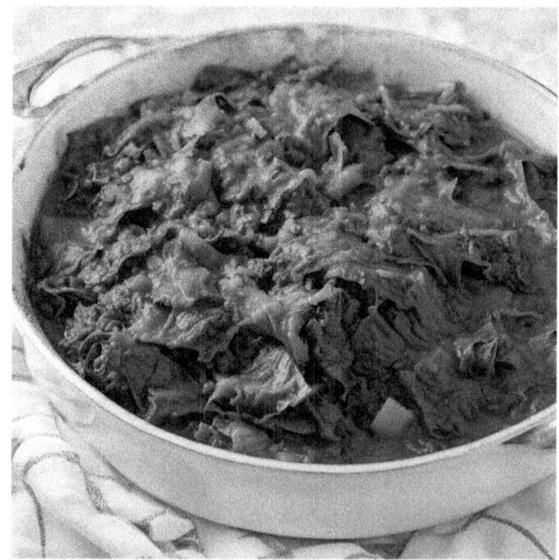

23. Turkish Shepherd's Salad

Ingredients (Serves 4)

- 2 large tomatoes, diced
- 1 cucumber, diced
- 1 green bell pepper, diced
- 1/2 red onion, finely chopped
- 1/4 cup fresh parsley, chopped
- 1/4 cup extra virgin olive oil
- 2 tablespoons fresh lemon juice
- 1 teaspoon dried mint
- 1/4 teaspoon ground black pepper

Instructions

1. Combine Vegetables: In a large bowl, combine the diced tomatoes, cucumber, green bell pepper, red onion, and parsley.
2. Make Dressing: In a small bowl, whisk together the olive oil, lemon juice, dried mint, and black pepper.
3. Toss Salad: Pour the dressing over the vegetables and toss gently to combine.
4. Serve: Serve immediately or chill for up to 1 hour to let the flavors meld.

Nutrition Information (Per Serving)

- Calories: 140 kcal
- Protein: 2g
- Carbohydrates: 10g
- Fiber: 3g
- Sugars: 5g (natural sugars from vegetables)
- Fat: 11g
- Saturated Fat: 1g
- Sodium: 20mg

Cooking Time

- **Preparation Time: 10 minutes**
- **Total Time: 10 minutes**

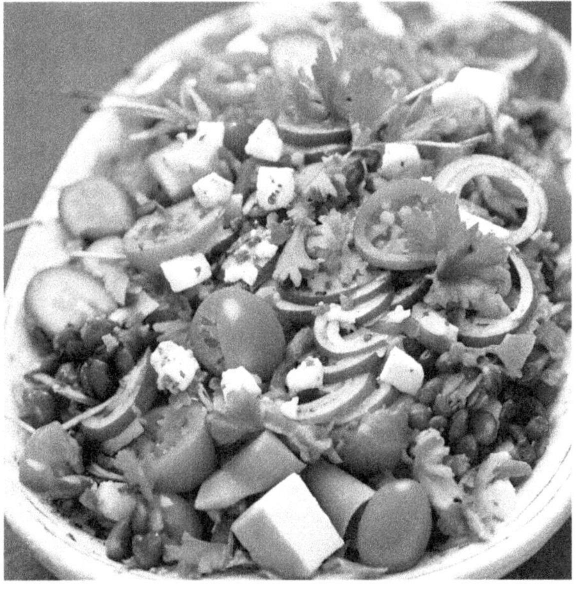

24. Chinese Garlic Green Beans

Ingredients (Serves 4)

- 1 pound green beans, trimmed
- 2 tablespoons extra virgin olive oil
- 4 cloves garlic, minced
- 1 tablespoon soy sauce (low-sodium)
- 1 teaspoon rice vinegar
- 1/4 teaspoon ground black pepper
- 1 tablespoon sesame seeds for garnish (optional)

Instructions

1. Blanch Green Beans: Bring a large pot of water to a boil. Add the green beans and cook for 2-3 minutes until just tender. Drain and rinse under cold water to stop the cooking process.
2. Heat Oil: In a large skillet or wok, heat the olive oil over medium-high heat. Add the minced garlic and cook for about 1 minute until fragrant.
3. Stir-Fry Green Beans: Add the blanched green beans to the skillet and stir-fry for 3-4 minutes until they begin to brown slightly.
4. Add Sauce: Stir in the soy sauce, rice vinegar, and black pepper. Cook for another 1-2 minutes until the beans are well coated and heated through.
5. Serve: Transfer to a serving dish and garnish with sesame seeds if desired. Serve warm.

Nutrition Information (Per Serving)

- Calories: 120 kcal
- Protein: 2g
- Carbohydrates: 10g
- Fiber: 4g
- Sugars: 3g (natural sugars from green beans)
- Fat: 8g
- Saturated Fat: 1g
- Sodium: 250mg

Cooking Time

- **Preparation Time: 5 minutes**
- **Cooking Time: 10 minutes**
- **Total Time: 15 minutes**

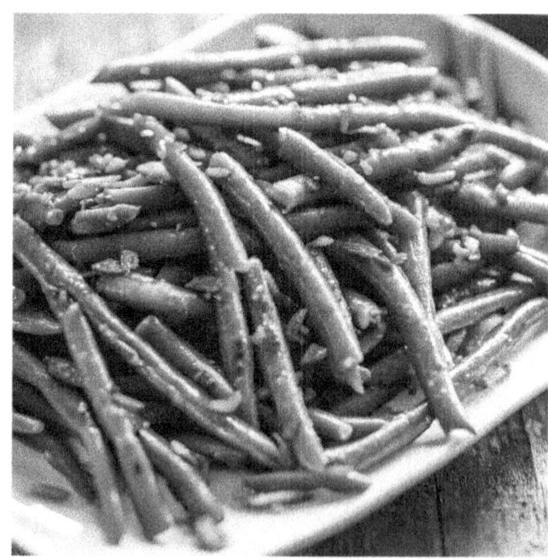

25. Greek Lemon Potatoes

Ingredients (Serves 4)

- 4 large potatoes, peeled and cut into wedges
- 1/4 cup extra virgin olive oil
- 1/4 cup fresh lemon juice
- 1 tablespoon dried oregano
- 1/4 teaspoon ground black pepper
- 1/2 cup low-sodium vegetable broth
- Fresh parsley for garnish (optional)

Instructions

1. Preheat Oven: Preheat your oven to 400°F (200°C). Grease a baking dish with a little olive oil.
2. Prepare Potatoes: Place the potato wedges in the baking dish. Drizzle with olive oil and lemon juice. Sprinkle with dried oregano and black pepper.
3. Add Broth: Pour the vegetable broth around the potatoes.
4. Bake: Bake in the preheated oven for 40-45 minutes, or until the potatoes are tender and golden brown, turning them halfway through.
5. Serve: Garnish with fresh parsley if desired and serve warm.

Nutrition Information (Per Serving)

- Calories: 250 kcal
- Protein: 4g
- Carbohydrates: 38g
- Fiber: 5g
- Sugars: 3g (natural sugars from potatoes)
- Fat: 10g
- Saturated Fat: 1g
- Sodium: 120mg

Cooking Time

- **Preparation Time: 10 minutes**
- **Cooking Time: 45 minutes**
- **Total Time: 55 minutes**

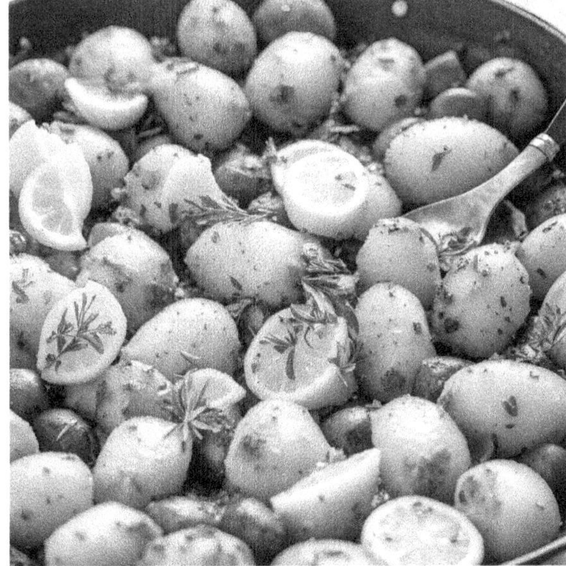

26. Spanish Grilled Vegetables with Romesco Sauce

Ingredients (Serves 4)

Grilled Vegetables:

- 1 zucchini, sliced into rounds
- 1 eggplant, sliced into rounds
- 1 red bell pepper, sliced into strips
- 1 yellow bell pepper, sliced into strips
- 1 red onion, sliced
- 2 tablespoons extra virgin olive oil
- 1/4 teaspoon ground black pepper

Romesco Sauce:

- 1/2 cup roasted red peppers, drained
- 1/4 cup blanched almonds
- 2 cloves garlic, minced
- 2 tablespoons extra virgin olive oil
- 1 tablespoon red wine vinegar
- 1 teaspoon smoked paprika
- 1/4 teaspoon ground black pepper

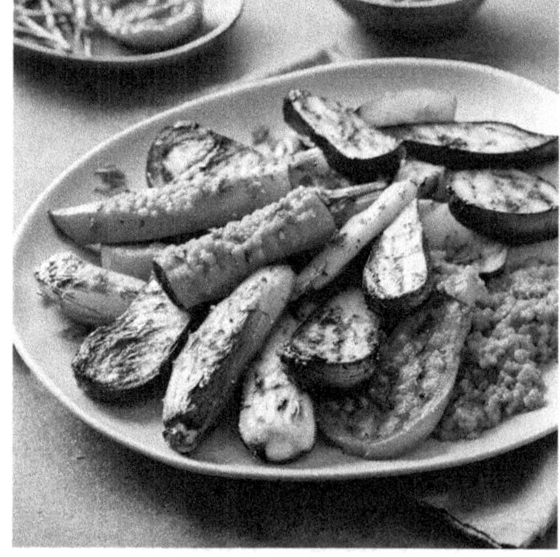

Instructions

1. Preheat Grill: Preheat your grill or grill pan to medium-high heat.
2. Prepare Vegetables: In a large bowl, toss the zucchini, eggplant, bell peppers, and red onion with olive oil and black pepper.
3. Grill Vegetables: Place the vegetables on the grill and cook for about 5-7 minutes, turning occasionally, until tender and have grill marks.
4. Make Romesco Sauce: While the vegetables are grilling, combine the roasted red peppers, almonds, garlic, olive oil, red wine vinegar, smoked paprika, and black pepper in a blender or food processor. Blend until smooth.
5. Serve: Arrange the grilled vegetables on a serving platter and serve with the Romesco sauce on the side.

Nutrition Information (Per Serving)

- Calories: 220 kcal   Protein: 4g   Carbohydrates: 14g   Fiber: 5g
- Sugars: 7g (natural sugars from vegetables)
- Fat: 16g   Saturated Fat: 2g   Sodium: 160m

Cooking Time

- **Preparation Time: 10 minutes**
- **Cooking Time: 10 minutes**
- **Total Time: 20 minutes**

Soup and Stew Recipes

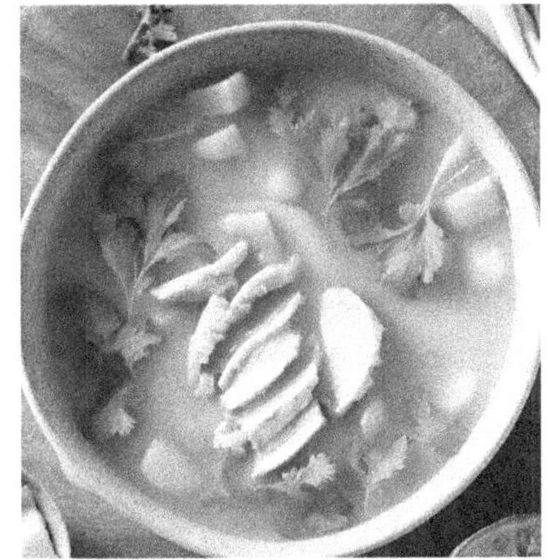

1. Turmeric Ginger Chicken Soup
Ingredients (Serves 4)
- 1 tablespoon extra virgin olive oil
- 1 onion, chopped
- 3 cloves garlic, minced
- 1 tablespoon fresh ginger, grated
- 1 teaspoon ground turmeric
- 1 pound boneless, skinless chicken breasts, cut into bite-sized pieces
- 4 cups low-sodium chicken broth
- 2 carrots, sliced
- 2 celery stalks, sliced
- 1 cup baby spinach
- 1 tablespoon fresh lemon juice
- 1/4 teaspoon ground black pepper
- Fresh parsley for garnish (optional)

Instructions
1. Heat Oil: In a large pot, heat the olive oil over medium heat. Add the onion and cook until softened, about 5 minutes.
2. Add Aromatics: Stir in the garlic, ginger, and turmeric, and cook for 1-2 minutes until fragrant.
3. Cook Chicken: Add the chicken pieces and cook for 5-7 minutes until they are no longer pink.
4. Add Broth and Vegetables: Pour in the chicken broth and add the carrots and celery. Bring to a boil, then reduce the heat and simmer for about 15 minutes until the vegetables are tender.
5. Add Spinach: Stir in the baby spinach and cook for another 2 minutes until wilted.
6. Finish Soup: Stir in the lemon juice and ground black pepper.
7. Serve: Garnish with fresh parsley if desired and serve warm.

Nutrition Information (Per Serving)
- Calories: 220 kcal Protein: 26g Carbohydrates: 10g
- Fiber: 3g
- Sugars: 4g (natural sugars from vegetables)
- Fat: 8g Saturated Fat: 1.5g Sodium: 350mg

Cooking Time
- **Preparation Time: 10 minutes**
- **Cooking Time: 30 minutes**
- **Total Time: 40 minutes**

2. Pumpkin and Sweet Potato Soup

Ingredients (Serves 4)

- 1 tablespoon extra virgin olive oil
- 1 onion, chopped
- 2 cloves garlic, minced
- 1 tablespoon fresh ginger, grated
- 2 cups pumpkin, peeled and cubed
- 2 cups sweet potatoes, peeled and cubed
- 4 cups low-sodium vegetable broth
- 1/2 teaspoon ground cinnamon
- 1/4 teaspoon ground black pepper
- 1/4 cup coconut milk (optional)
- Fresh cilantro for garnish (optional)

Instructions

1. Heat Oil: In a large pot, heat the olive oil over medium heat. Add the onion and cook until softened, about 5 minutes.
2. Add Garlic and Ginger: Stir in the garlic and ginger, and cook for 1-2 minutes until fragrant.
3. Add Vegetables and Broth: Add the pumpkin and sweet potatoes to the pot. Pour in the vegetable broth and bring to a boil.
4. Simmer: Reduce the heat and simmer for about 20 minutes until the vegetables are tender.
5. Blend Soup: Using an immersion blender or regular blender, puree the soup until smooth.
6. Season: Stir in the ground cinnamon, black pepper, and coconut milk if using.
7. Serve: Garnish with fresh cilantro if desired and serve warm.

Nutrition Information (Per Serving)

- Calories: 180 kcal
- Protein: 3g
- Carbohydrates: 34g
- Fiber: 7g
- Sugars: 9g (natural sugars from vegetables)
- Fat: 5g
- Saturated Fat: 2g
- Sodium: 320mg

Cooking Time

- **Preparation Time: 10 minutes**
- **Cooking Time: 25 minutes**
- **Total Time: 35 minutes**

3. Vegetable and Barley Soup
Ingredients (Serves 4)

- 1 tablespoon extra virgin olive oil
- 1 onion, chopped
- 2 cloves garlic, minced
- 2 carrots, sliced
- 2 celery stalks, sliced
- 1 zucchini, diced
- 1 cup mushrooms, sliced
- 1/2 cup barley
- 4 cups low-sodium vegetable broth
- 1 can (14.5 ounces) diced tomatoes, no salt added
- 1 teaspoon dried thyme
- 1/4 teaspoon ground black pepper
- 2 cups spinach, chopped
- Fresh parsley for garnish (optional)

Instructions

1. Heat Oil: In a large pot, heat the olive oil over medium heat. Add the onion and cook until softened, about 5 minutes.
2. Add Garlic and Vegetables: Stir in the garlic, carrots, celery, zucchini, and mushrooms. Cook for about 5 minutes until the vegetables start to soften.
3. Add Barley and Broth: Add the barley, vegetable broth, diced tomatoes, dried thyme, and black pepper. Bring to a boil.
4. Simmer: Reduce the heat and simmer for about 30 minutes until the barley is tender.
5. Add Spinach: Stir in the chopped spinach and cook for another 2-3 minutes until wilted.
6. Serve: Garnish with fresh parsley if desired and serve warm.

Nutrition Information (Per Serving)

- Calories: 220 kcal Protein: 6g Carbohydrates: 40g Fiber: 9g
- Sugars: 10g (natural sugars from vegetables)
- Fat: 6g Saturated Fat: 1g Sodium: 320mg

Cooking Time

- **Preparation Time: 10 minutes**
- **Cooking Time: 35 minutes**
- **Total Time: 45 minutes**

4. Moroccan Chickpea and Tomato Stew

Ingredients (Serves 4)

- 1 tablespoon extra virgin olive oil
- 1 onion, chopped
- 2 cloves garlic, minced
- 1 tablespoon fresh ginger, grated
- 1 teaspoon ground cumin
- 1 teaspoon ground coriander
- 1 teaspoon smoked paprika
- 1/2 teaspoon ground cinnamon
- 1/4 teaspoon ground black pepper
- 1 can (14.5 ounces) chickpeas, rinsed and drained
- 1 can (14.5 ounces) diced tomatoes, no salt added
- 2 cups low-sodium vegetable broth
- 2 cups spinach, chopped
- 1 tablespoon fresh lemon juice
- Fresh cilantro for garnish (optional)

Instructions

1. Heat Oil: In a large pot, heat the olive oil over medium heat. Add the onion and cook until softened, about 5 minutes.
2. Add Garlic and Spices: Stir in the garlic, ginger, cumin, coriander, smoked paprika, cinnamon, and black pepper. Cook for 1-2 minutes until fragrant.
3. Add Chickpeas and Tomatoes: Add the chickpeas and diced tomatoes to the pot. Pour in the vegetable broth and bring to a boil.
4. Simmer: Reduce the heat and simmer for about 20 minutes until the flavors meld together.
5. Add Spinach: Stir in the chopped spinach and cook for another 2-3 minutes until wilted.
6. Finish Stew: Stir in the lemon juice.
7. Serve: Garnish with fresh cilantro if desired and serve warm.

Nutrition Information (Per Serving)

- Calories: 200 kcal   Protein: 7g Carbohydrates: 32g
- Fiber: 9g
- Sugars: 9g (natural sugars from vegetables)
- Fat: 6g   Saturated Fat: 1g   Sodium: 320mg

Cooking Time

- **Preparation Time: 10 minutes**
- **Cooking Time: 25 minutes**
- **Total Time: 35 minutes**

5. Minestrone with Pesto

Ingredients (Serves 4)

- 1 tablespoon extra virgin olive oil
- 1 onion, chopped
- 2 cloves garlic, minced
- 2 carrots, diced
- 2 celery stalks, diced
- 1 zucchini, diced
- 1 can (14.5 ounces) diced tomatoes, no salt added
- 4 cups low-sodium vegetable broth
- 1 cup cooked cannellini beans
- 1/2 cup pasta (gluten-free or whole grain)
- 1 teaspoon dried oregano
- 1/4 teaspoon ground black pepper
- 2 cups spinach, chopped
- 1/4 cup fresh basil pesto (store-bought or homemade)
- Fresh basil for garnish (optional)

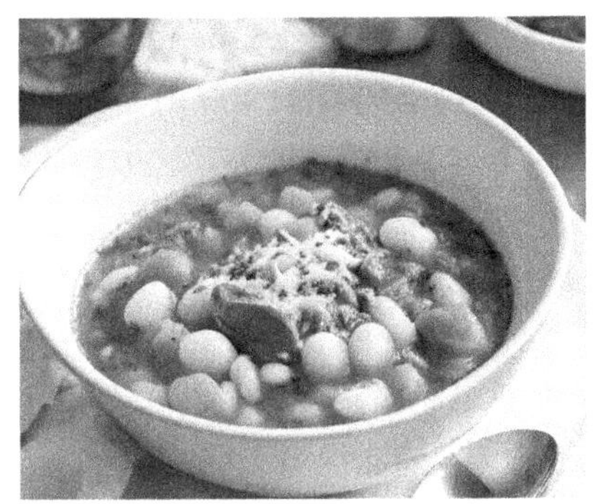

Instructions

1. Heat Oil: In a large pot, heat the olive oil over medium heat. Add the onion and cook until softened, about 5 minutes.
2. Add Garlic and Vegetables: Stir in the garlic, carrots, celery, and zucchini. Cook for about 5 minutes until the vegetables start to soften.
3. Add Tomatoes and Broth: Add the diced tomatoes and vegetable broth to the pot. Stir in the cannellini beans, pasta, dried oregano, and black pepper. Bring to a boil.
4. Simmer: Reduce the heat and simmer for about 15 minutes until the pasta is cooked and the vegetables are tender.
5. Add Spinach: Stir in the chopped spinach and cook for another 2 minutes until wilted.
6. Serve with Pesto: Ladle the minestrone into bowls and top each serving with a spoonful of basil pesto. Garnish with fresh basil if desired and serve warm.

Nutrition Information (Per Serving)

- Calories: 280 kcal   Protein: 9g   Carbohydrates: 40g   Fiber: 8g
- Sugars: 10g (natural sugars from vegetables)
- Fat: 10g   Saturated Fat: 2g   Sodium: 360mg

Cooking Time

- **Preparation Time: 10 minutes**
- **Cooking Time: 25 minutes**
- **Total Time: 35 minutes**

6. Thai Coconut Soup (Tom Kha Gai)
Ingredients (Serves 4)

- 1 tablespoon extra virgin olive oil
- 1 onion, chopped
- 2 cloves garlic, minced
- 1 tablespoon fresh ginger, grated
- 2 stalks lemongrass, chopped
- 1 pound boneless, skinless chicken breasts, thinly sliced
- 4 cups low-sodium chicken broth
- 1 can (14 ounces) coconut milk (light or full-fat)
- 1 cup mushrooms, sliced
- 1 red bell pepper, sliced
- 2 tablespoons fish sauce (or soy sauce for a vegetarian option)
- 1 tablespoon fresh lime juice
- 1/4 teaspoon ground black pepper
- 1/4 cup fresh cilantro, chopped
- 1 red chili, sliced for garnish (optional)

Instructions

1. Heat Oil: In a large pot, heat the olive oil over medium heat. Add the onion and cook until softened, about 5 minutes.
2. Add Garlic and Aromatics: Stir in the garlic, ginger, and lemongrass. Cook for 1-2 minutes until fragrant.
3. Cook Chicken: Add the thinly sliced chicken and cook for about 5 minutes until it starts to turn opaque.
4. Add Broth and Coconut Milk: Pour in the chicken broth and coconut milk. Bring to a simmer.
5. Add Vegetables: Stir in the mushrooms and red bell pepper. Cook for about 10 minutes until the vegetables are tender and the chicken is fully cooked.
6. Finish Soup: Stir in the fish sauce, lime juice, and black pepper.
7. Serve: Garnish with fresh cilantro and red chili slices if desired. Serve warm.

Nutrition Information (Per Serving)

- Calories: 300 kcal Protein: 20g Carbohydrates: 12g Fiber: 3g
- Sugars: 5g (natural sugars from vegetables)
- Fat: 20g Saturated Fat: 12g Sodium: 400mg

Cooking Time

- **Preparation Time: 10 minutes**
- **Cooking Time: 25 minutes**
- **Total Time: 35 minutes**

7. Black Bean Soup with Cilantro

Ingredients (Serves 4)

- 1 tablespoon extra virgin olive oil
- 1 onion, chopped
- 3 cloves garlic, minced
- 1 red bell pepper, chopped
- 2 cans (15 ounces each) black beans, rinsed and drained
- 4 cups low-sodium vegetable broth
- 1 teaspoon ground cumin
- 1 teaspoon smoked paprika
- 1/4 teaspoon ground black pepper
- 1/4 cup fresh cilantro, chopped
- 1 tablespoon fresh lime juice
- Optional toppings: diced avocado, chopped green onions, and extra cilantro

Instructions

1. Heat Oil: In a large pot, heat the olive oil over medium heat. Add the onion and cook until softened, about 5 minutes.
2. Add Garlic and Bell Pepper: Stir in the garlic and red bell pepper, and cook for 3-4 minutes until the pepper begins to soften.
3. Add Beans and Broth: Add the black beans, vegetable broth, cumin, smoked paprika, and black pepper. Bring to a boil, then reduce the heat and simmer for about 20 minutes.
4. Blend Soup: Using an immersion blender, partially blend the soup to thicken it, leaving some beans whole for texture.
5. Finish Soup: Stir in the fresh cilantro and lime juice.
6. Serve: Ladle the soup into bowls and top with diced avocado, chopped green onions, and extra cilantro if desired. Serve warm.

Nutrition Information (Per Serving)

- Calories: 210 kcal Protein: 10g Carbohydrates: 35g Fiber: 12g
- Sugars: 5g (natural sugars from vegetables)
- Fat: 5g Saturated Fat: 0.5g Sodium: 400mg

Cooking Time

- **Preparation Time: 10 minutes**
- **Cooking Time: 25 minutes**
- **Total Time: 35 minutes**

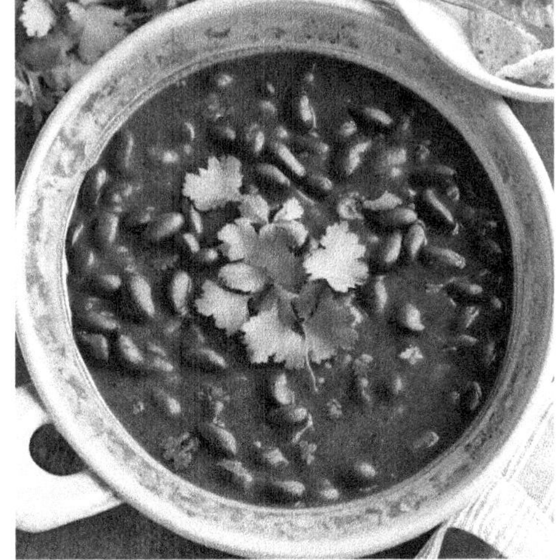

8. Chinese Hot and Sour Soup
Ingredients (Serves 4)
- 1 tablespoon extra virgin olive oil
- 1 onion, thinly sliced
- 2 cloves garlic, minced
- 1 tablespoon fresh ginger, grated
- 4 cups low-sodium vegetable broth
- 1 cup shiitake mushrooms, sliced
- 1 cup bamboo shoots, julienned
- 1/2 cup firm tofu, cubed
- 1/4 cup rice vinegar
- 2 tablespoons soy sauce (low-sodium)
- 1 tablespoon chili paste (adjust to taste)
- 1/4 teaspoon ground black pepper
- 2 tablespoons cornstarch mixed with 2 tablespoons water
- 2 green onions, chopped for garnish
- 1/4 cup fresh cilantro, chopped for garnish

Instructions
1. Heat Oil: In a large pot, heat the olive oil over medium heat. Add the onion and cook until softened, about 5 minutes.
2. Add Garlic and Ginger: Stir in the garlic and ginger, and cook for 1-2 minutes until fragrant.
3. Add Broth and Vegetables: Pour in the vegetable broth and add the mushrooms, bamboo shoots, and tofu. Bring to a boil.
4. Season: Stir in the rice vinegar, soy sauce, chili paste, and black pepper. Simmer for about 10 minutes.
5. Thicken Soup: Stir in the cornstarch mixture and cook for another 2-3 minutes until the soup thickens slightly.
6. Serve: Ladle the soup into bowls and garnish with chopped green onions and fresh cilantro. Serve warm.

Nutrition Information (Per Serving)
- Calories: 150 kcal Protein: 5g Carbohydrates: 16g Fiber: 3g
- Sugars: 4g (natural sugars from vegetables)
- Fat: 6g Saturated Fat: 1g Sodium: 500mg

Cooking Time
- **Preparation Time: 10 minutes**
- **Cooking Time: 20 minutes**
- **Total Time: 30 minutes**

9. Lebanese Lentil Soup (Shorbat Adas)
Ingredients (Serves 4)
* 1 tablespoon extra virgin olive oil
* 1 onion, chopped
* 2 cloves garlic, minced
* 1 cup red lentils, rinsed
* 4 cups low-sodium vegetable broth
* 1 teaspoon ground cumin
* 1/2 teaspoon ground coriander
* 1/4 teaspoon ground black pepper
* 1/2 teaspoon turmeric powder
* 1 large carrot, diced
* 1 potato, diced
* 1/4 cup fresh lemon juice
* Fresh parsley for garnish (optional)

Instructions
1. Heat Oil: In a large pot, heat the olive oil over medium heat. Add the onion and cook until softened, about 5 minutes.
2. Add Garlic and Spices: Stir in the garlic, cumin, coriander, black pepper, and turmeric. Cook for 1-2 minutes until fragrant.
3. Add Lentils and Vegetables: Add the red lentils, diced carrot, and potato to the pot. Pour in the vegetable broth and bring to a boil.
4. Simmer: Reduce the heat and simmer for about 20-25 minutes until the lentils and vegetables are tender.
5. Blend Soup: Using an immersion blender, partially blend the soup to thicken it, leaving some chunks for texture.
6. Finish Soup: Stir in the fresh lemon juice.
7. Serve: Garnish with fresh parsley if desired and serve warm.

Nutrition Information (Per Serving)
* Calories: 200 kcal Protein: 9g   Carbohydrates: 33g
* Fiber: 10g
* Sugars: 5g (natural sugars from vegetables)
* Fat: 5g Saturated Fat: 1g Sodium: 320mg

Cooking Time
* **Preparation Time: 10 minutes**
* **Cooking Time: 25 minutes**
* **Total Time: 35 minutes**

10. African Peanut Stew

Ingredients (Serves 4)

- 1 tablespoon extra virgin olive oil
- 1 onion, chopped
- 3 cloves garlic, minced
- 1 tablespoon fresh ginger, grated
- 1 red bell pepper, diced
- 2 sweet potatoes, peeled and cubed
- 1 can (14.5 ounces) diced tomatoes, no salt added
- 4 cups low-sodium vegetable broth
- 1/2 cup natural peanut butter
- 1 teaspoon ground cumin
- 1/4 teaspoon ground black pepper
- 1/4 teaspoon red pepper flakes
- 1 cup spinach, chopped
- 1/4 cup fresh cilantro, chopped
- Fresh lime wedges for serving (optional)

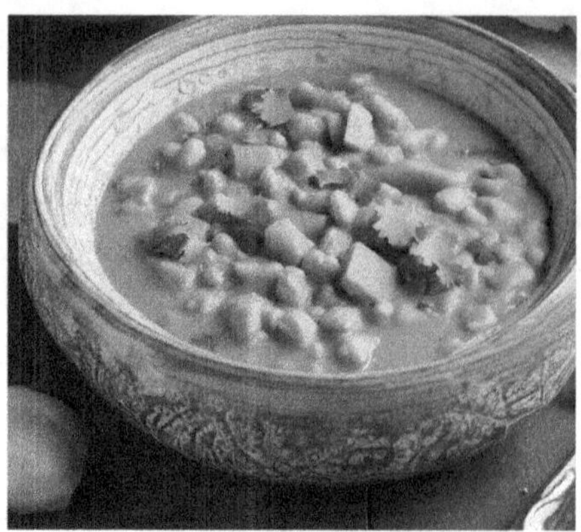

Instructions

1. Heat Oil: In a large pot, heat the olive oil over medium heat. Add the onion and cook until softened, about 5 minutes.
2. Add Garlic and Ginger: Stir in the garlic and ginger, and cook for 1-2 minutes until fragrant.
3. Add Vegetables and Broth: Add the red bell pepper, sweet potatoes, diced tomatoes, and vegetable broth. Bring to a boil.
4. Add Peanut Butter and Spices: Stir in the peanut butter, ground cumin, black pepper, and red pepper flakes. Reduce the heat and simmer for about 20 minutes until the sweet potatoes are tender.
5. Add Spinach: Stir in the chopped spinach and cook for another 2-3 minutes until wilted.
6. Serve: Garnish with fresh cilantro and serve with lime wedges if desired.

Nutrition Information (Per Serving)

- Calories: 300 kcal Protein: 9g Carbohydrates: 38g   Fiber: 8g
- Sugars: 9g (natural sugars from vegetables)
- Fat: 15g Saturated Fat: 3g Sodium: 350mg

Cooking Time

- **Preparation Time: 10 minutes**
- **Cooking Time: 25 minutes**
- **Total Time: 35 minutes**

11. Italian Ribollita

Ingredients (Serves 4)

- 2 tablespoons extra virgin olive oil
- 1 onion, chopped
- 2 cloves garlic, minced
- 2 carrots, diced
- 2 celery stalks, diced
- 1 zucchini, diced
- 1 can (14.5 ounces) diced tomatoes, no salt added
- 4 cups low-sodium vegetable broth
- 1 can (14.5 ounces) cannellini beans, rinsed and drained
- 1/4 teaspoon ground black pepper
- 1/4 teaspoon red pepper flakes
- 2 cups kale, chopped
- 4 slices day-old whole grain bread, cubed
- Fresh basil for garnish (optional)

Instructions

1. Heat Oil: In a large pot, heat the olive oil over medium heat. Add the onion and cook until softened, about 5 minutes.
2. Add Garlic and Vegetables: Stir in the garlic, carrots, celery, and zucchini. Cook for about 5 minutes until the vegetables start to soften.
3. Add Tomatoes and Broth: Add the diced tomatoes and vegetable broth. Stir in the cannellini beans, black pepper, and red pepper flakes. Bring to a boil.
4. Add Kale and Bread: Reduce the heat and add the chopped kale and bread cubes. Simmer for about 10 minutes until the bread breaks down and the soup thickens.
5. Serve: Garnish with fresh basil if desired and serve warm.

Nutrition Information (Per Serving)

- Calories: 280 kcal Protein: 10g Carbohydrates: 45g   Fiber: 10g
- Sugars: 8g (natural sugars from vegetables)
- Fat: 7g Saturated Fat: 1g   Sodium: 400mg

Cooking Time

- **Preparation Time: 10 minutes**
- **Cooking Time: 25 minutes**
- **Total Time: 35 minutes**

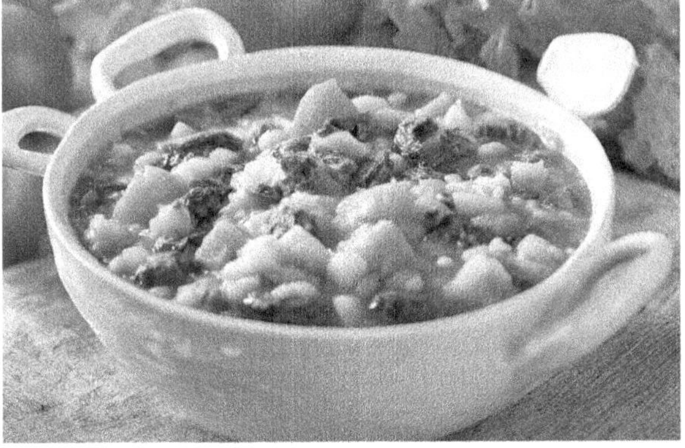

12. Peruvian Quinoa and Vegetable Soup

Ingredients (Serves 4)

- 1 tablespoon extra virgin olive oil
- 1 onion, chopped
- 2 cloves garlic, minced
- 1 cup quinoa, rinsed
- 4 cups low-sodium vegetable broth
- 1 large carrot, diced
- 1 zucchini, diced
- 1 cup corn kernels (fresh or frozen)
- 1 cup green beans, chopped
- 1 teaspoon ground cumin
- 1/4 teaspoon ground black pepper
- 1/4 cup fresh cilantro, chopped
- 1 tablespoon fresh lime juice

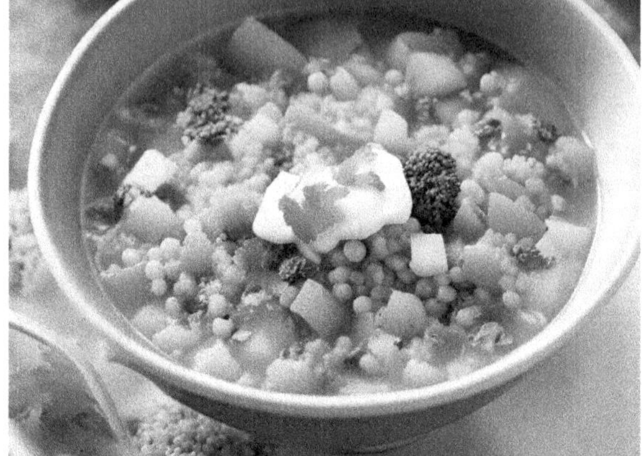

Instructions

1. Heat Oil: In a large pot, heat the olive oil over medium heat. Add the onion and cook until softened, about 5 minutes.
2. Add Garlic and Quinoa: Stir in the garlic and quinoa, and cook for 1-2 minutes until the quinoa is lightly toasted.
3. Add Broth and Vegetables: Pour in the vegetable broth and add the carrot, zucchini, corn, and green beans. Bring to a boil.
4. Simmer: Reduce the heat and simmer for about 20 minutes until the quinoa and vegetables are tender.
5. Season: Stir in the ground cumin, black pepper, cilantro, and lime juice.
6. Serve: Serve warm.

Nutrition Information (Per Serving)

- Calories: 250 kcal Protein: 8g Carbohydrates: 40g
- Fiber: 8g
- Sugars: 7g (natural sugars from vegetables)
- Fat: 7g Saturated Fat: 1g Sodium: 350mg

Cooking Time

- **Preparation Time: 10 minutes**
- **Cooking Time: 20 minutes**
- **Total Time: 30 minutes**

13. Hungarian Mushroom Soup

Ingredients (Serves 4)

- 2 tablespoons extra virgin olive oil
- 1 onion, chopped
- 2 cloves garlic, minced
- 1 pound mushrooms, sliced
- 1 tablespoon paprika
- 1 teaspoon dried thyme
- 1/4 teaspoon ground black pepper
- 4 cups low-sodium vegetable broth
- 1 cup unsweetened almond milk (or any other non-dairy milk)
- 2 tablespoons fresh lemon juice
- 1/4 cup fresh dill, chopped

Instructions

1. Heat Oil: In a large pot, heat the olive oil over medium heat. Add the onion and cook until softened, about 5 minutes.
2. Add Garlic and Mushrooms: Stir in the garlic and mushrooms. Cook for about 10 minutes until the mushrooms release their juices and start to brown.
3. Add Spices: Stir in the paprika, thyme, and black pepper. Cook for another 2 minutes until fragrant.
4. Add Broth and Milk: Pour in the vegetable broth and almond milk. Bring to a simmer and cook for about 10 minutes.
5. Finish Soup: Stir in the lemon juice and fresh dill.
6. Serve: Serve warm.

Nutrition Information (Per Serving)

- Calories: 150 kcal
- Protein: 5g
- Carbohydrates: 16g
- Fiber: 4g
- Sugars: 6g (natural sugars from vegetables)
- Fat: 8g
- Saturated Fat: 1g
- Sodium: 300mg

Cooking Time

- **Preparation Time: 10 minutes**
- **Cooking Time: 25 minutes**
- **Total Time: 35 minutes**

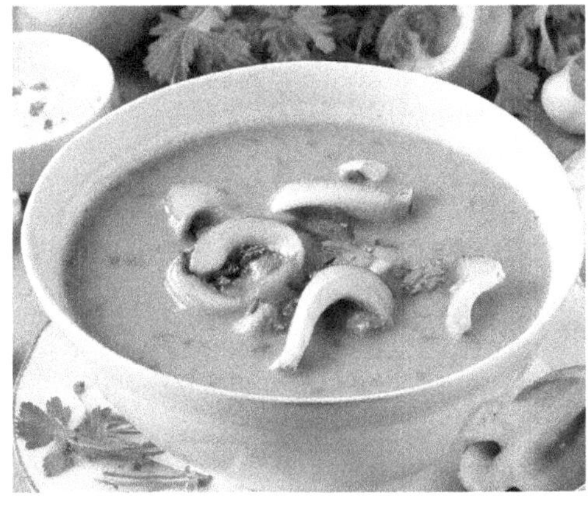

14. Portuguese Kale Soup (Caldo Verde)

Ingredients (Serves 4)

- 1 tablespoon extra virgin olive oil
- 1 onion, chopped
- 2 cloves garlic, minced
- 1 pound potatoes, peeled and diced
- 4 cups low-sodium vegetable broth
- 4 cups kale, chopped
- 1/4 teaspoon ground black pepper
- 1/4 teaspoon red pepper flakes
- Fresh lemon wedges for serving (optional)

Instructions

1. Heat Oil: In a large pot, heat the olive oil over medium heat. Add the onion and cook until softened, about 5 minutes.
2. Add Garlic and Potatoes: Stir in the garlic and potatoes. Cook for another 5 minutes until the potatoes start to soften.
3. Add Broth: Pour in the vegetable broth and bring to a boil.
4. Simmer: Reduce the heat and simmer for about 15 minutes until the potatoes are tender.
5. Blend Soup: Using an immersion blender, partially blend the soup to thicken it, leaving some chunks for texture.
6. Add Kale and Spices: Stir in the chopped kale, black pepper, and red pepper flakes. Cook for another 5 minutes until the kale is tender.
7. Serve: Serve warm with fresh lemon wedges if desired.

Nutrition Information (Per Serving)

- Calories: 180 kcal
- Protein: 5g
- Carbohydrates: 30g
- Fiber: 6g
- Sugars: 5g (natural sugars from vegetables)
- Fat: 6g
- Saturated Fat: 1g
- Sodium: 300mg

Cooking Time

- **Preparation Time: 10 minutes**
- **Cooking Time: 25 minutes**
- **Total Time: 35 minutes**

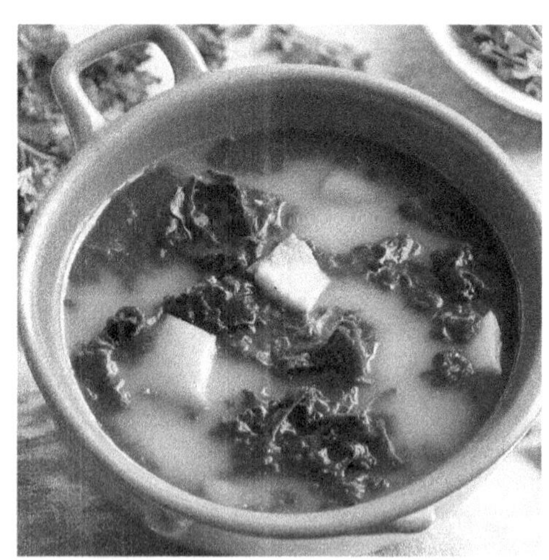

15. West African Groundnut Stew

Ingredients (Serves 4)

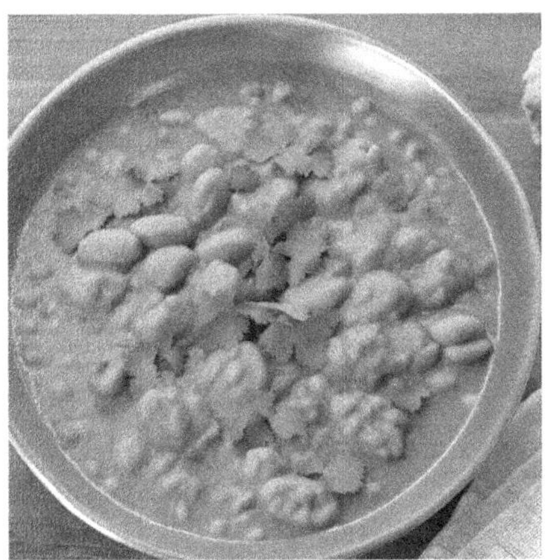

- 1 tablespoon extra virgin olive oil
- 1 onion, chopped
- 3 cloves garlic, minced
- 1 tablespoon fresh ginger, grated
- 1 red bell pepper, diced
- 2 sweet potatoes, peeled and cubed
- 1 can (14.5 ounces) diced tomatoes, no salt added
- 4 cups low-sodium vegetable broth
- 1/2 cup natural peanut butter
- 1 teaspoon ground cumin
- 1/4 teaspoon ground black pepper
- 1/4 teaspoon cayenne pepper (optional)
- 1 cup spinach, chopped
- 1/4 cup fresh cilantro, chopped
- Fresh lime wedges for serving (optional)

Instructions

1. Heat Oil: In a large pot, heat the olive oil over medium heat. Add the onion and cook until softened, about 5 minutes.
2. Add Garlic and Ginger: Stir in the garlic and ginger, and cook for 1-2 minutes until fragrant.
3. Add Vegetables and Broth: Add the red bell pepper, sweet potatoes, diced tomatoes, and vegetable broth. Bring to a boil.
4. Add Peanut Butter and Spices: Stir in the peanut butter, ground cumin, black pepper, and cayenne pepper (if using). Reduce the heat and simmer for about 20 minutes until the sweet potatoes are tender.
5. Add Spinach: Stir in the chopped spinach and cook for another 2-3 minutes until wilted.
6. Serve: Garnish with fresh cilantro and serve with lime wedges if desired.

Nutrition Information (Per Serving)

- Calories: 320 kcal
- Protein: 9g
- Carbohydrates: 38g
- Fiber: 8g
- Sugars: 10g (natural sugars from vegetables)
- Fat: 16g
- Saturated Fat: 3g
- Sodium: 350mg

Cooking Time

- **Preparation Time: 10 minutes**
- **Cooking Time: 25 minutes**
- **Total Time: 35 minutes**

16. Vietnamese Sweet Potato and Kale Soup
Ingredients (Serves 4)

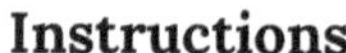

- 1 tablespoon extra virgin olive oil
- 1 onion, chopped
- 3 cloves garlic, minced
- 1 tablespoon fresh ginger, grated
- 2 sweet potatoes, peeled and cubed
- 4 cups low-sodium vegetable broth
- 1 tablespoon soy sauce (low-sodium)
- 1/4 teaspoon ground black pepper
- 2 cups kale, chopped
- 1/4 cup fresh cilantro, chopped
- 1 tablespoon fresh lime juice

Instructions

1. Heat Oil: In a large pot, heat the olive oil over medium heat. Add the onion and cook until softened, about 5 minutes.
2. Add Garlic and Ginger: Stir in the garlic and ginger, and cook for 1-2 minutes until fragrant.
3. Add Sweet Potatoes and Broth: Add the sweet potatoes and vegetable broth. Bring to a boil.
4. Simmer: Reduce the heat and simmer for about 20 minutes until the sweet potatoes are tender.
5. Season and Add Kale: Stir in the soy sauce, black pepper, and chopped kale. Cook for another 5 minutes until the kale is tender.
6. Finish Soup: Stir in the fresh cilantro and lime juice.
7. Serve: Serve warm.

Nutrition Information (Per Serving)

- Calories: 200 kcal
- Protein: 4g
- Carbohydrates: 34g
- Fiber: 7g
- Sugars: 10g (natural sugars from vegetables)
- Fat: 7g
- Saturated Fat: 1g
- Sodium: 350mg

Cooking Time

- **Preparation Time: 10 minutes**
- **Cooking Time: 25 minutes**
- **Total Time: 35 minutes**

17. Middle Eastern Lentil and Eggplant Stew

Ingredients (Serves 4)

- 1 tablespoon extra virgin olive oil
- 1 onion, chopped
- 3 cloves garlic, minced
- 1 eggplant, diced
- 1 cup red lentils, rinsed
- 1 can (14.5 ounces) diced tomatoes, no salt added
- 4 cups low-sodium vegetable broth
- 1 teaspoon ground cumin
- 1 teaspoon ground coriander
- 1/4 teaspoon ground black pepper
- 1/4 teaspoon ground cinnamon
- 1/4 cup fresh parsley, chopped
- 1 tablespoon fresh lemon juice

Instructions

1. Heat Oil: In a large pot, heat the olive oil over medium heat. Add the onion and cook until softened, about 5 minutes.
2. Add Garlic and Eggplant: Stir in the garlic and eggplant. Cook for about 5 minutes until the eggplant begins to soften.
3. Add Lentils and Spices: Add the red lentils, diced tomatoes, vegetable broth, ground cumin, ground coriander, black pepper, and ground cinnamon. Bring to a boil.
4. Simmer: Reduce the heat and simmer for about 25 minutes until the lentils and eggplant are tender.
5. Finish Stew: Stir in the fresh parsley and lemon juice.
6. Serve: Serve warm.

Nutrition Information (Per Serving)

- Calories: 250 kcal
- Protein: 10g
- Carbohydrates: 40g
- Fiber: 12g
- Sugars: 10g (natural sugars from vegetables)
- Fat: 7g
- Saturated Fat: 1g
- Sodium: 320mg

Cooking Time

- **Preparation Time: 10 minutes**
- **Cooking Time: 25 minutes**
- **Total Time: 35 minutes**

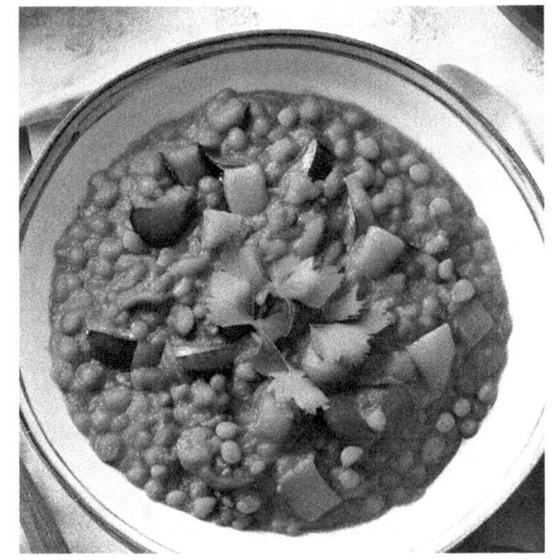

18. Spanish Saffron Vegetable Stew

Ingredients (Serves 4)

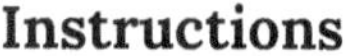

- 1 tablespoon extra virgin olive oil
- 1 onion, chopped
- 2 cloves garlic, minced
- 1 red bell pepper, chopped
- 1 zucchini, diced
- 1 cup green beans, chopped
- 1 can (14.5 ounces) diced tomatoes, no salt added
- 4 cups low-sodium vegetable broth
- 1/2 teaspoon saffron threads
- 1 teaspoon smoked paprika
- 1/4 teaspoon ground black pepper
- 1/4 cup fresh parsley, chopped
- 1 tablespoon fresh lemon juice

Instructions

1. Heat Oil: In a large pot, heat the olive oil over medium heat. Add the onion and cook until softened, about 5 minutes.
2. Add Garlic and Bell Pepper: Stir in the garlic and red bell pepper. Cook for 3-4 minutes until the pepper begins to soften.
3. Add Vegetables and Spices: Add the zucchini, green beans, diced tomatoes, vegetable broth, saffron threads, smoked paprika, and black pepper. Bring to a boil.
4. Simmer: Reduce the heat and simmer for about 20 minutes until the vegetables are tender.
5. Finish Stew: Stir in the fresh parsley and lemon juice.
6. Serve: Serve warm.

Nutrition Information (Per Serving)

- Calories: 200 kcal
- Protein: 5g
- Carbohydrates: 32g
- Fiber: 8g
- Sugars: 10g (natural sugars from vegetables)
- Fat: 7g
- Saturated Fat: 1g
- Sodium: 320mg

Cooking Time

- **Preparation Time: 10 minutes**
- **Cooking Time: 20 minutes**
- **Total Time: 30 minutes**

19. Italian Escarole and Bean Soup
Ingredients (Serves 4)

- 1 tablespoon extra virgin olive oil
- 1 onion, chopped
- 3 cloves garlic, minced
- 1 head escarole, chopped
- 1 can (14.5 ounces) cannellini beans, rinsed and drained
- 4 cups low-sodium vegetable broth
- 1/4 teaspoon ground black pepper
- 1/4 teaspoon red pepper flakes (optional)
- 1/4 cup fresh parsley, chopped
- 1 tablespoon fresh lemon juice

Instructions

1. Heat Oil: In a large pot, heat the olive oil over medium heat. Add the onion and cook until softened, about 5 minutes.
2. Add Garlic: Stir in the garlic and cook for 1-2 minutes until fragrant.
3. Add Escarole and Beans: Add the chopped escarole and cannellini beans. Cook for about 5 minutes until the escarole begins to wilt.
4. Add Broth and Spices: Pour in the vegetable broth, black pepper, and red pepper flakes (if using). Bring to a boil.
5. Simmer: Reduce the heat and simmer for about 10 minutes until the escarole is tender.
6. Finish Soup: Stir in the fresh parsley and lemon juice.
7. Serve: Serve warm.

Nutrition Information (Per Serving)

- Calories: 180 kcal
- Protein: 7g
- Carbohydrates: 28g
- Fiber: 8g
- Sugars: 4g (natural sugars from vegetables)
- Fat: 6g
- Saturated Fat: 1g
- Sodium: 320mg

Cooking Time

- **Preparation Time: 10 minutes**
- **Cooking Time: 15 minutes**
- **Total Time: 25 minutes**

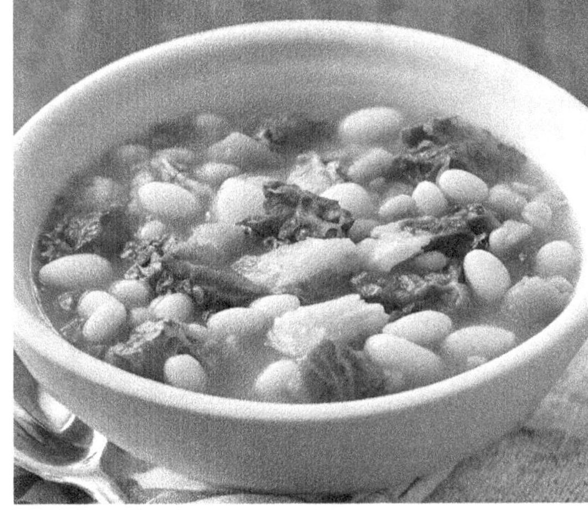

20. Mexican Pozole Verde

Ingredients (Serves 4)

- 1 tablespoon extra virgin olive oil
- 1 onion, chopped
- 3 cloves garlic, minced
- 1 pound boneless, skinless chicken breasts, cubed
- 4 cups low-sodium chicken broth
- 1 can (14.5 ounces) hominy, rinsed and drained
- 2 cups tomatillos, husked and chopped
- 2 poblano peppers, seeded and chopped
- 1/4 cup fresh cilantro, chopped
- 1 teaspoon ground cumin
- 1/4 teaspoon ground black pepper
- 1 tablespoon fresh lime juice
- Optional toppings: sliced radishes, shredded cabbage, chopped avocado

Instructions

1. Heat Oil: In a large pot, heat the olive oil over medium heat. Add the onion and cook until softened, about 5 minutes.
2. Add Garlic and Chicken: Stir in the garlic and chicken cubes. Cook for about 5 minutes until the chicken is browned.
3. Add Broth and Vegetables: Add the chicken broth, hominy, tomatillos, and poblano peppers. Bring to a boil.
4. Simmer: Reduce the heat and simmer for about 20 minutes until the chicken is cooked through and the vegetables are tender.
5. Blend Soup: Using an immersion blender, partially blend the soup to thicken it slightly, leaving some chunks for texture.
6. Finish Soup: Stir in the fresh cilantro, ground cumin, black pepper, and lime juice.
7. Serve: Serve warm with optional toppings like sliced radishes, shredded cabbage, and chopped avocado.

Nutrition Information (Per Serving)

- Calories: 300 kcal
- Protein: 25g
- Carbohydrates: 30g
- Fiber: 6g
- Sugars: 7g (natural sugars from vegetables)
- Fat: 10g
- Saturated Fat: 1.5g
- Sodium: 400mg

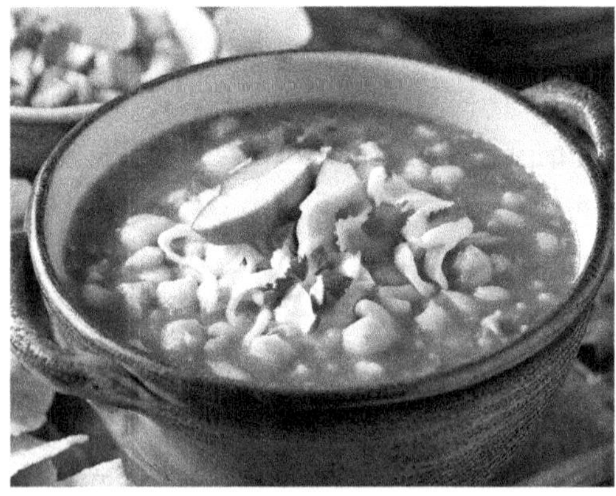

Cooking Time

- **Preparation Time: 10 minutes**
- **Cooking Time: 25 minutes**
- **Total Time: 35 minutes**

21. Mediterranean White Bean Soup

Ingredients (Serves 4)

- 2 tablespoons extra virgin olive oil
- 1 onion, chopped
- 3 cloves garlic, minced
- 2 carrots, diced
- 2 celery stalks, diced
- 1 can (14.5 ounces) diced tomatoes, no salt added
- 4 cups low-sodium vegetable broth
- 2 cans (15 ounces each) white beans, rinsed and drained
- 1 teaspoon dried oregano
- 1 teaspoon dried thyme
- 1/4 teaspoon ground black pepper
- 2 cups kale, chopped
- 1/4 cup fresh parsley, chopped
- 1 tablespoon fresh lemon juice

Instructions

1. Heat Oil: In a large pot, heat the olive oil over medium heat. Add the onion and cook until softened, about 5 minutes.
2. Add Garlic and Vegetables: Stir in the garlic, carrots, and celery. Cook for another 5 minutes until the vegetables start to soften.
3. Add Tomatoes and Broth: Add the diced tomatoes and vegetable broth. Bring to a boil.
4. Add Beans and Spices: Stir in the white beans, oregano, thyme, and black pepper. Reduce the heat and simmer for about 20 minutes.
5. Add Kale: Stir in the chopped kale and cook for another 5 minutes until the kale is tender.
6. Finish Soup: Stir in the fresh parsley and lemon juice.
7. Serve: Serve warm.

Nutrition Information (Per Serving)

- Calories: 220 kcal
- Protein: 10g
- Carbohydrates: 35g
- Fiber: 9g
- Sugars: 6g (natural sugars from vegetables)
- Fat: 6g
- Saturated Fat: 1g
- Sodium: 320mg

Cooking Time

- **Preparation Time: 10 minutes**
- **Cooking Time: 25 minutes**
- **Total Time: 35 minutes**

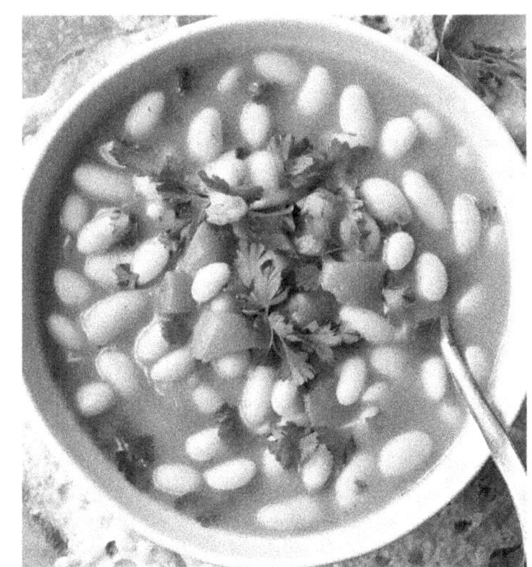

22. Filipino Mung Bean Soup (Monggo Guisado)
Ingredients (Serves 4)

- 1 cup mung beans, rinsed
- 6 cups water
- 2 tablespoons extra virgin olive oil
- 1 onion, chopped
- 3 cloves garlic, minced
- 1 tomato, chopped
- 1 cup spinach, chopped
- 1/4 teaspoon ground black pepper
- 1 tablespoon fish sauce (optional, or use soy sauce for a vegetarian option)
- 1/4 cup fresh cilantro, chopped

Instructions

1. Cook Mung Beans: In a large pot, combine the mung beans and water. Bring to a boil, then reduce the heat and simmer for about 30 minutes until the beans are tender. Drain and set aside.
2. Heat Oil: In a separate large pot, heat the olive oil over medium heat. Add the onion and cook until softened, about 5 minutes.
3. Add Garlic and Tomato: Stir in the garlic and tomato. Cook for another 3-4 minutes until the tomato begins to soften.
4. Combine Beans and Vegetables: Add the cooked mung beans to the pot. Stir in the spinach, black pepper, and fish sauce (or soy sauce).
5. Simmer: Simmer for another 10 minutes until the spinach is wilted and the flavors meld together.
6. Finish Soup: Stir in the fresh cilantro.
7. Serve: Serve warm.

Nutrition Information (Per Serving)

- Calories: 180 kcal
- Protein: 9g
- Carbohydrates: 29g
- Fiber: 7g
- Sugars: 3g (natural sugars from vegetables)
- Fat: 5g
- Saturated Fat: 1g
- Sodium: 280mg

Cooking Time

- **Preparation Time: 10 minutes**
- **Total Time: 40 minutes**

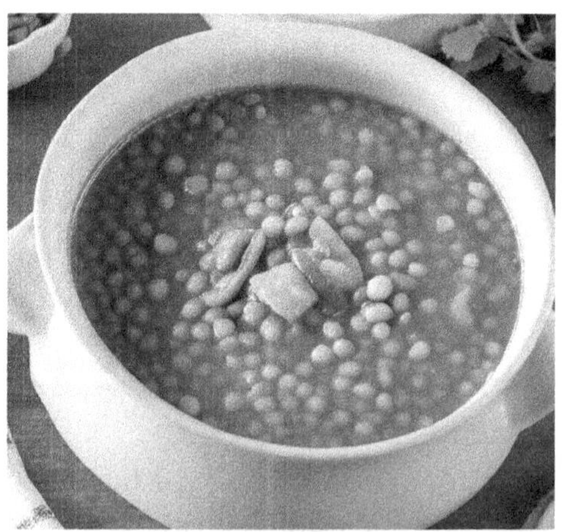

23. Japanese Udon Noodle Soup

Ingredients (Serves 4)

- 8 ounces dried udon noodles
- 1 tablespoon extra virgin olive oil
- 1 onion, thinly sliced
- 3 cloves garlic, minced
- 1 tablespoon fresh ginger, grated
- 4 cups low-sodium vegetable broth
- 4 cups water
- 1/4 cup low-sodium soy sauce
- 1 cup shiitake mushrooms, sliced
- 1 cup bok choy, chopped
- 1 carrot, julienned
- 1/4 teaspoon ground black pepper
- 2 green onions, sliced for garnish
- 1 tablespoon sesame seeds for garnish (optional)

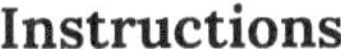

Instructions

1. Cook Udon Noodles: Cook the udon noodles according to the package instructions. Drain and set aside.
2. Heat Oil: In a large pot, heat the olive oil over medium heat. Add the onion and cook until softened, about 5 minutes.
3. Add Garlic and Ginger: Stir in the garlic and ginger, and cook for 1-2 minutes until fragrant.
4. Add Broth and Water: Pour in the vegetable broth and water. Bring to a simmer.
5. Add Vegetables and Soy Sauce: Stir in the soy sauce, shiitake mushrooms, bok choy, carrot, and black pepper. Simmer for about 10 minutes until the vegetables are tender.
6. Combine Noodles and Broth: Add the cooked udon noodles to the pot and heat through.
7. Serve: Ladle the soup into bowls and garnish with sliced green onions and sesame seeds if desired. Serve warm.

Nutrition Information (Per Serving)

- Calories: 250 kcal Protein: 7g Carbohydrates: 45g Fiber: 4g
- Sugars: 5g (natural sugars from vegetables)
- Fat: 6g Saturated Fat: 1g Sodium: 480mg

Cooking Time

- **Preparation Time: 10 minutes**
- **Cooking Time: 20 minutes**
- **Total Time: 30 minutes**

10-WEEK MEAL PLAN

Week 1
Monday
- Breakfast: Oatmeal with Berries and Nuts
- Lunch: Mediterranean Quinoa Salad
- Dinner: Baked Salmon with Lemon and Dill

Tuesday
- Breakfast: Avocado Toast with Cherry Tomatoes
- Lunch: Thai Green Curry with Vegetables
- Dinner: Grilled Tuna Steaks with Avocado Salsa

Wednesday
- Breakfast: Greek Yogurt with Honey and Almonds
- Lunch: Moroccan Carrot Salad
- Dinner: Shrimp and Quinoa Salad

Thursday
- Breakfast: Banana and Chia Seed Pudding
- Lunch: Indian Spiced Cauliflower
- Dinner: Garlic Butter Shrimp

Friday
- Breakfast: Smoothie Bowl with Spinach and Pineapple
- Lunch: Chinese Stir-Fried Bok Choy
- Dinner: Miso Glazed Cod

Saturday
- Breakfast: Buckwheat Pancakes with Fresh Fruit
- Lunch: Lebanese Tabbouleh
- Dinner: Seared Scallops with Spinach

Sunday
- Breakfast: Quinoa Breakfast Bowl with Almond Butter
- Lunch: Korean Bibimbap with Vegetables
- Dinner: Mediterranean Baked Halibut

Week 2
Monday
- Breakfast: Apple and Cinnamon Overnight Oats
- Lunch: Vietnamese Fresh Spring Rolls
- Dinner: Lemon Herb Grilled Shrimp

Tuesday
- Breakfast: Sweet Potato Hash with Kale
- Lunch: Turkish Eggplant Imam Bayildi
- Dinner: Salmon and Asparagus Foil Packets

Wednesday
- Breakfast: Almond Flour Muffins with Blueberries
- Lunch: Ethiopian Lentil Stew (Misir Wot)
- Dinner: Tuna Salad with White Beans and Arugula

Thursday
- Breakfast: Mango and Turmeric Smoothie
- Lunch: Middle Eastern Roasted Vegetables
- Dinner: Spicy Baked Cod

Friday
- Breakfast: Cottage Cheese with Pineapple and Walnuts
- Lunch: Caribbean Callaloo
- Dinner: Garlic Lemon Shrimp Pasta

Saturday
- Breakfast: Green Tea and Berry Smoothie
- Lunch: Argentinian Chimichurri Vegetables
- Dinner: Citrus Marinated Salmon

Sunday
- Breakfast: Millet Porridge with Almonds and Raisins
- Lunch: Greek Briam (Roasted Vegetables)
- Dinner: Grilled Mahi Mahi with Mango Salsa

Week 3

Monday
- Breakfast: Egg White Omelette with Bell Peppers and Onions
- Lunch: Moroccan Zaalouk (Eggplant Dip)
- Dinner: Salmon and Sweet Potato Cakes

Tuesday
- Breakfast: Chia and Flaxseed Porridge
- Lunch: Peruvian Quinoa and Vegetable Stew
- Dinner: Steamed Mussels with Garlic and Parsley

Wednesday
- Breakfast: Baked Apples with Cinnamon and Walnuts
- Lunch: Italian Caponata
- Dinner: Tuna and Avocado Salad

Thursday
- Breakfast: Lentil Breakfast Bowl with Spinach
- Lunch: Mexican Grilled Vegetable Tacos
- Dinner: Baked Sole with Lemon and Capers

Friday
- Breakfast: Pumpkin and Oat Breakfast Bars
- Lunch: Lebanese Tabbouleh
- Dinner: Lemon Dill Baked Haddock

Saturday
- Breakfast: Smoked Salmon and Avocado Toast
- Lunch: Korean Spicy Stir-Fried Vegetables (Kimchi Bokkeum)
- Dinner: Tuna and Olive Tapenade Wraps

Sunday
- Breakfast: Berry and Almond Smoothie
- Lunch: Indian Spinach and Potato (Aloo Palak)
- Dinner: Ginger Soy Glazed Salmon

Week 4

Monday
- Breakfast: Mixed Nut and Fruit Breakfast Bowl
- Lunch: Chinese Garlic Green Beans
- Dinner: Broiled Lemon Garlic Fish

Tuesday
- Breakfast: Quinoa and Blueberry Breakfast Parfait
- Lunch: Greek Lemon Potatoes
- Dinner: Shrimp and Zucchini Noodles

Wednesday
- Breakfast: Pumpkin Seed and Apple Muesli
- Lunch: Spanish Grilled Vegetables with Romesco Sauce
- Dinner: Baked Trout with Almonds

Thursday
- Breakfast: Turmeric Ginger Chicken Soup
- Lunch: Ethiopian Stewed Collard Greens
- Dinner: Clam and Kale Soup

Friday
- Breakfast: Pumpkin and Sweet Potato Soup
- Lunch: Italian Panzanella Salad
- Dinner: Baked Tilapia with Tomatoes and Basil

Saturday
- Breakfast: Vegetable and Barley Soup
- Lunch: Vietnamese Lemongrass Tofu with Vegetables
- Dinner: Shrimp and Avocado Rice Bowls

Sunday
- Breakfast: Moroccan Chickpea and Tomato Stew
- Lunch: Turkish Shepherd's Salad
- Dinner: Tuna and Chickpea Salad

Week 5

Monday
- Breakfast: Minestrone with Pesto
- Lunch: Chinese Hot and Sour Soup
- Dinner: Broiled Sardines with Lemon and Herbs

Tuesday
- Breakfast: Thai Coconut Soup (Tom Kha Gai)
- Lunch: Peruvian Quinoa and Vegetable Soup
- Dinner: Grilled Swordfish with Pineapple Salsa

Wednesday
- Breakfast: Black Bean Soup with Cilantro
- Lunch: Argentinian Vegetable Stew (Locro)
- Dinner: Salmon and Asparagus Foil Packets

Thursday
- Breakfast: Filipino Mung Bean Soup (Monggo Guisado)
- Lunch: Japanese Udon Noodle Soup
- Dinner: Tuna and Avocado Salad

Friday
- Breakfast: Hungarian Mushroom Soup
- Lunch: West African Groundnut Stew
- Dinner: Lemon Dill Baked Haddock

Saturday
- Breakfast: Portuguese Kale Soup (Caldo Verde)
- Lunch: Middle Eastern Lentil and Eggplant Stew
- Dinner: Spicy Baked Cod

Sunday
- Breakfast: Mediterranean White Bean Soup
- Lunch: Vietnamese Sweet Potato and Kale Soup
- Dinner: Broiled Lemon Garlic Fish

Week 6

Monday
- Breakfast: Millet Porridge with Almonds and Raisins
- Lunch: Greek Lemon Potatoes
- Dinner: Seared Scallops with Spinach

Tuesday
- Breakfast: Green Tea and Berry Smoothie
- Lunch: Italian Caponata
- Dinner: Shrimp and Avocado Rice Bowls

Wednesday
- Breakfast: Smoked Salmon and Avocado Toast
- Lunch: Turkish Eggplant Imam Bayildi
- Dinner: Baked Trout with Almonds

Thursday
- Breakfast: Pumpkin and Oat Breakfast Bars
- Lunch: Korean Bibimbap with Vegetables
- Dinner: Lemon Herb Grilled Shrimp

Friday
- Breakfast: Apple and Cinnamon Overnight Oats
- Lunch: Chinese Garlic Green Beans
- Dinner: Broiled Lemon Garlic Fish

Saturday
- Breakfast: Smoothie Bowl with Spinach and Pineapple
- Lunch: Ethiopian Lentil Stew (Misir Wot)
- Dinner: Grilled Swordfish with Pineapple Salsa

Sunday
- Breakfast: Egg White Omelette with Bell Peppers and Onions
- Lunch: Caribbean Callaloo
- Dinner: Salmon and Sweet Potato Cakes

Week 7

Monday
- Breakfast: Quinoa and Blueberry Breakfast Parfait
- Lunch: Moroccan Carrot Salad
- Dinner: Garlic Lemon Shrimp Pasta

Tuesday
- Breakfast: Mango and Turmeric Smoothie
- Lunch: Vietnamese Lemongrass Tofu with Vegetables
- Dinner: Grilled Tuna Steaks with Avocado Salsa

Wednesday
- Breakfast: Mixed Nut and Fruit Breakfast Bowl
- Lunch: Chinese Stir-Fried Bok Choy
- Dinner: Mediterranean Baked Halibut

Thursday
- Breakfast: Cottage Cheese with Pineapple and Walnuts
- Lunch: Middle Eastern Roasted Vegetables
- Dinner: Tuna Salad with White Beans and Arugula

Friday

- Breakfast: Berry and Almond Smoothie
- Lunch: Indian Spiced Cauliflower
- Dinner: Miso Glazed Cod

Saturday

- Breakfast: Millet Porridge with Almonds and Raisins
- Lunch: Lebanese Tabbouleh
- Dinner: Citrus Marinated Salmon

Sunday

- Breakfast: Greek Yogurt with Honey and Almonds
- Lunch: Spanish Saffron Vegetable Stew
- Dinner: Tuna and Olive Tapenade Wraps

Week 8

Monday

- Breakfast: Pumpkin and Sweet Potato Soup
- Lunch: Korean Spicy Stir-Fried Vegetables (Kimchi Bokkeum)
- Dinner: Broiled Sardines with Lemon and Herbs

Tuesday

- Breakfast: Baked Apples with Cinnamon and Walnuts
- Lunch: Italian Panzanella Salad
- Dinner: Ginger Soy Glazed Salmon

Wednesday

- Breakfast: Lentil Breakfast Bowl with Spinach
- Lunch: Vietnamese Fresh Spring Rolls
- Dinner: Shrimp and Zucchini Noodles

Thursday

- Breakfast: Chia and Flaxseed Porridge
- Lunch: Turkish Shepherd's Salad
- Dinner: Baked Sole with Lemon and Capers

Friday

- Breakfast: Black Bean Soup with Cilantro
- Lunch: Mexican Grilled Vegetable Tacos
- Dinner: Garlic Butter Shrimp

Saturday

- Breakfast: Cottage Cheese with Pineapple and Walnuts
- Lunch: Caribbean Callaloo
- Dinner: Grilled Swordfish with Pineapple Salsa

Sunday

- Breakfast: Egg White Omelette with Bell Peppers and Onions
- Lunch: Ethiopian Stewed Collard Greens
- Dinner: Lemon Dill Baked Haddock

Week 9

Monday

- Breakfast: Apple and Cinnamon Overnight Oats
- Lunch: Argentinian Chimichurri Vegetables
- Dinner: Steamed Mussels with Garlic and Parsley

Tuesday

- Breakfast: Quinoa Breakfast Bowl with Almond Butter
- Lunch: Italian Escarole and Bean Soup
- Dinner: Spicy Baked Cod

Wednesday

- Breakfast: Mixed Nut and Fruit Breakfast Bowl
- Lunch: Vietnamese Sweet Potato and Kale Soup
- Dinner: Broiled Lemon Garlic Fish

Thursday

- Breakfast: Greek Yogurt with Honey and Almonds
- Lunch: Indian Spinach and Potato (Aloo Palak)
- Dinner: Shrimp and Avocado Rice Bowls

Friday

- Breakfast: Mango and Turmeric Smoothie
- Lunch: Middle Eastern Lentil and Eggplant Stew
- Dinner: Grilled Tuna Steaks with Avocado Salsa

Saturday

- Breakfast: Green Tea and Berry Smoothie
- Lunch: Greek Briam (Roasted Vegetables)
- Dinner: Baked Tilapia with Tomatoes and Basil

Sunday

- Breakfast: Millet Porridge with Almonds and Raisins
- Lunch: Chinese Hot and Sour Soup
- Dinner: Garlic Lemon Shrimp Pasta

Week 10

Monday

- Breakfast: Smoked Salmon and Avocado Toast
- Lunch: Peruvian Quinoa and Vegetable Stew
- Dinner: Grilled Mahi Mahi with Mango Salsa

Tuesday
- Breakfast: Almond Flour Muffins with Blueberries
- Lunch: Spanish Grilled Vegetables with Romesco Sauce
- Dinner: Salmon and Sweet Potato Cakes

Wednesday
- Breakfast: Buckwheat Pancakes with Fresh Fruit
- Lunch: Argentinian Vegetable Stew (Locro)
- Dinner: Seared Scallops with Spinach

Thursday
- Breakfast: Sweet Potato Hash with Kale
- Lunch: Caribbean Callaloo
- Dinner: Baked Trout with Almonds

Friday
- Breakfast: Black Bean Soup with Cilantro
- Lunch: Korean Bibimbap with Vegetables
- Dinner: Tuna and Olive Tapenade Wraps

Saturday
- Breakfast: Smoothie Bowl with Spinach and Pineapple
- Lunch: Ethiopian Lentil Stew (Misir Wot)
- Dinner: Garlic Butter Shrimp

Sunday
- Breakfast: Chia and Flaxseed Porridge
- Lunch: Mexican Pozole Verde
- Dinner: Broiled Sardines with Lemon and Herbs

WEEKLY MEAL PLANNER + WORKBOOK

	BREAKFAST	LUNCH	DINNER	SNACKS
MONDAY				
TUESDAY				
WEDNESDAY				
THURSDAY				
FRIDAY				
SATURDAY				
SUNDAY				

What are your primary goals for following the arthritis diet? List at least three.

WEEKLY MEAL PLANNER + WORKBOOK

	BREAKFAST	LUNCH	DINNER	SNACKS
MONDAY				
TUESDAY				
WEDNESDAY				
THURSDAY				
FRIDAY				
SATURDAY				
SUNDAY				

How do you hope the arthritis diet will improve your overall health and well-being?

WEEKLY MEAL PLANNER + WORKBOOK

	BREAKFAST	LUNCH	DINNER	SNACKS
MONDAY				
TUESDAY				
WEDNESDAY				
THURSDAY				
FRIDAY				
SATURDAY				
SUNDAY				

Describe your current eating habits. How often do you eat vegetables, fruits, and whole grains?

WEEKLY MEAL PLANNER + WORKBOOK

	BREAKFAST	LUNCH	DINNER	SNACKS
MONDAY				
TUESDAY				
WEDNESDAY				
THURSDAY				
FRIDAY				
SATURDAY				
SUNDAY				

What are your most common arthritis symptoms? How do they affect your daily life?

WEEKLY MEAL PLANNER + WORKBOOK

	BREAKFAST	LUNCH	DINNER	SNACKS
MONDAY				
TUESDAY				
WEDNESDAY				
THURSDAY				
FRIDAY				
SATURDAY				
SUNDAY				

Have you noticed any foods that seem to worsen your arthritis symptoms? List them.

WEEKLY MEAL PLANNER + WORKBOOK

	BREAKFAST	LUNCH	DINNER	SNACKS
MONDAY				
TUESDAY				
WEDNESDAY				
THURSDAY				
FRIDAY				
SATURDAY				
SUNDAY				

Plan a typical arthritis-friendly breakfast. What ingredients will you use?

WEEKLY MEAL PLANNER + WORKBOOK

	BREAKFAST	LUNCH	DINNER	SNACKS
MONDAY				
TUESDAY				
WEDNESDAY				
THURSDAY				
FRIDAY				
SATURDAY				
SUNDAY				

What challenges do you anticipate in meal planning for the arthritis diet? How can you overcome them?

....

....

....

....

....

....

WEEKLY MEAL PLANNER + WORKBOOK

	BREAKFAST	LUNCH	DINNER	SNACKS
MONDAY				
TUESDAY				
WEDNESDAY				
THURSDAY				
FRIDAY				
SATURDAY				
SUNDAY				

Describe a new recipe you'd like to try. What excites you about it?

WEEKLY MEAL PLANNER + WORKBOOK

	BREAKFAST	LUNCH	DINNER	SNACKS
MONDAY				
TUESDAY				
WEDNESDAY				
THURSDAY				
FRIDAY				
SATURDAY				
SUNDAY				

How do you plan to incorporate physical activity into your routine to complement your new diet?

WEEKLY MEAL PLANNER + WORKBOOK

	BREAKFAST	LUNCH	DINNER	SNACKS
MONDAY				
TUESDAY				
WEDNESDAY				
THURSDAY				
FRIDAY				
SATURDAY				
SUNDAY				

What types of exercises do you enjoy, and how can you adapt them for your arthritis?

WEEKLY MEAL PLANNER + WORKBOOK

	BREAKFAST	LUNCH	DINNER	SNACKS
MONDAY				
TUESDAY				
WEDNESDAY				
THURSDAY				
FRIDAY				
SATURDAY				
SUNDAY				

Who can you rely on for support as you start the arthritis diet? How will they help you?

WEEKLY MEAL PLANNER + WORKBOOK

	BREAKFAST	LUNCH	DINNER	SNACKS
MONDAY				
TUESDAY				
WEDNESDAY				
THURSDAY				
FRIDAY				
SATURDAY				
SUNDAY				

- **Are there any supplements you're considering adding to your diet? Why?**

WEEKLY MEAL PLANNER + WORKBOOK

	BREAKFAST	LUNCH	DINNER	SNACKS
MONDAY				
TUESDAY				
WEDNESDAY				
THURSDAY				
FRIDAY				
SATURDAY				
SUNDAY				

Write a personal commitment statement for your arthritis diet journey. What promises are you making to yourself?

Scan the QR code below to get a surprise bonus!